Thrombolytic therapy for acute myocardial infarction

Contributors and members
of the Prairie Cardiovascular Center
Springfield, Illinois

James T. Dove MD
David P. Hamm MD
Richard E. Katholi MD
Deborah L. Koester BSN
Brian D. Miller MD
H. Weston Moses MD
Joel A. Schneider MD
Harry A. Wellons MD
Robert C. Woodruff MD
W.T. Woods Jr. PhD

Thrombolytic therapy for acute myocardial infarction

GEORGE J. TAYLOR MD
Clinical Associate Professor of Medicine
Southern Illinois University School of Medicine
Springfield, Illinois

BOSTON

BLACKWELL SCIENTIFIC PUBLICATIONS
OXFORD LONDON EDINBURGH
MELBOURNE PARIS BERLIN VIENNA

© 1992 by
Blackwell Scientific Publications, Inc.
Editorial offices:
3 Cambridge Center, Cambridge
  Massachusetts 02142, USA
Osney Mead, Oxford OX2 0EL,
  England
25 John Street, London WC1N 2BL
  England
23 Ainslie Place, Edinburgh EH3 6AJ
  Scotland
54 University Street, Carlton Victoria
  3053, Australia

Other editorial offices:
Librairie Arnette SA
2, rue Casimir-Delavigne
75006 Paris
France

Blackwell Wissenschafts-Verlag
Meinekestrasse 4
D-1000 Berlin 15
Germany

Blackwell MZV
Feldgasse 13
A-1238 Wien
Austria

First published 1992

Set by Excel Typesetters Company,
Hong Kong
Printed and bound in the
United States of America
by Maple-Vail, New York

92   93   94   95   5   4   3   2   1

DISTRIBUTORS

USA
  Blackwell Scientific Publications, Inc.
  3 Cambridge Center
  Cambridge, Massachusetts 02142
  (*Orders*: Tel: 800 759-6102
              617 225-0401)

Canada
  Times Mirror Professional
  Publishing, Ltd
  5240 Finch Avenue East
  Scarborough, Ontario M1S 5A2
  (*Orders*: Tel: 800 268-4178
              416 298-1588)

Australia
  Blackwell Scientific Publications
  (Australia) Pty Ltd
  54 University Street
  Carlton, Victoria 3053
  (*Orders*: Tel: 03 347-0300)

Outside North America and Australia
  Marston Book Services Ltd
  PO Box 87
  Oxford OX2 0DT
  (*Orders*: Tel: 0865 791155
             Fax: 0865 791927
             Telex: 837515)

Library of Congress
Cataloguing-in-Publication Data

Taylor, George Jesse.
    Thrombolytic therapy for
  acute myocardial infarction/
  George J. Taylor.
          p.   cm.
    Includes bibliographical references
  and index.
    ISBN 0-86542-200-1
    1. Myocardial infarction—
  Chemotherapy.
    2. Fibrinolytic agents.
    I. Title.
    [DNLM: 1. Myocardial infarction
  —drug therapy.
    2. Thrombolytic Therapy.
  WG 300 T241t]
  RC685.I6T39   1992
  616.1′237061—dc20
  DNLM/DLC

This last decade has been a fine time to practice cardiology in rural Illinois. Developing a strategy for thrombolytic therapy in the primary care setting has been exciting, satisfying work. We gratefully dedicate this book to our colleagues in central Illinois, the nursing staff in their community hospitals, and our excellent nursing staff at St John's Hospital, all of whom pioneered the use of thrombolytic therapy at the grass roots level.

Contents

Preface

This book is a curriculum for doctors and nurses who treat patients suffering from acute MI. Treatment of acute MI used to be easier for the health care team, as the immediate diagnosis was not as critical as it is now. There was little we could do to change the MI process itself, and our primary goal was to treat its complications. The most important step was getting the patient with possible MI on a cardiac monitor in order to detect VF. The emergency room staff could thus initiate treatment even if unable to interpret the ECG. It made no difference to prognosis if the diagnosis of MI was not confirmed until the next day. This was usually accomplished when enzyme results were available and the ECG interpretation arrived from a remote ECG reading facility.

All that has changed with the introduction of thrombolytic therapy. Now the immediate diagnosis of MI is a medical necessity, as thrombolytic therapy must be applied promptly to be effective. The best predictor of myocardial salvage is early thrombolysis. A patient treated within 1 hour of onset of chest pain will have the best clinical result. Those treated at 3 hours will do fairly well, but with variable results. Patients treated after 3 hours have far less opportunity for salvage of muscle. The first doctor who sees and treats the patient has the greatest opportunity to change the outcome of MI by making a diagnosis and initiating therapy.

Thrombolytic therapy does save lives and does lower the morbidity of acute MI. Simply put, to treat patients with acute MI competently, you must be able to use thrombolytic therapy.

This book is not designed for use merely as a reference. Instead, we at the Prairie Cardiovascular Center hope you will read it through, probably in a couple of evenings. We hope to give you and your emergency department and CCU staff the facts needed to use thrombolytic therapy, to devise a subsequent treatment strategy, and to treat common problems seen with acute MI and with thrombolysis.

We have helped treat over 2000 patients with thrombolytic therapy for acute MI since 1981. Most of these patients had therapy initiated by doctors in small community hospitals in central Illinois, and we know that emergency department and primary care physicians can safely and effectively use thrombolytic drugs. We commonly reference our published clinical work. The approach we describe reflects this large experience, and we freely admit that it describes our point of view. The book will also provide information from clinical trials that have answered practical questions about application of this new treatment approach. But it is not a literature review. We speak to you from the vantage point of having a hands-on experience with this powerful new therapeutic modality.

I appreciate the forebearance of my wife, Marilyn, during the preparation of this manuscript. I am also grateful for the secretarial assistance of Brenda Ruyle and for the artwork done by Bernardine A. Hatcher, Thomas P. Broad, Linda Ragel, and Charles S. Kilbourne. The editorial assistance of Owsly Gillespie of Springfield and Victoria Reeders and Michael Snider at Blackwell Scientific Publications is greatly appreciated.

List of abbreviations

aPTT	Activated partial thromboplastin time
APSAC	Anisoylated plasminogen streptokinase activator complex
BBB	Bundle branch block
CCU	Coronary care unit
CHF	Congestive heart failure
CK	Creatine kinase
CNS	Central nervous system
ECG	Electrocardiogram
GI	Gastrointestinal
GU	Genitourinary
ICU	Intensive care unit
LV	Left ventricular
LVEF	Left ventricular ejection fraction
MI	Myocardial infarction
RNA	Radionuclide angiogram
rt-PA	Recombinant tissue plasminogen activator
RV	Right ventricular
STK	Streptokinase
t-PA	Tissue plasminogen activator
UK	Urokinase
VF	Ventricular fibrillation
VT	Ventricular tachycardia

Notice The indications and dosages of all drugs in this book have been recommended in the medical literature and conform to the practices of the general medical community. The medications described do not necessarily have specific approval by the Food and Drug Administration (FDA) for use in the diseases and dosages for which they are recommended. The package insert for each drug should be consulted for use and dosage as approved by the FDA. Because standards for usage change, it is advisable to keep abreast of revised recommendations, particularly those concerning new drugs.

Thrombolytic therapy for acute myocardial infarction

Chapter 1

A rationale for thrombolytic therapy in your hospital

No doubt about it, in the 1990s you must be able to use thrombolytic therapy if you treat patients with acute MI. This is especially true if you are the first doctor to evaluate the patient. It is in the patient's best interest that the first doctor is the treating doctor. After occlusion of the coronary artery, heart muscle death is progressive with time. For patients with chest pain the clock is ticking, and with each quarter hour that passes, there is irreversible death of myocardium. The patient in the emergency room really does not have time to wait for the cardiologist to arrive, or time to transfer to another facility for consultation.

This chapter will review evidence documenting efficacy of thrombolytic therapy. The clinical studies that are most useful for this purpose are those which randomly allocated patients to treatment with thrombolytic drugs or placebo. For a more formal review of the individual trials, a summary is provided in Appendix 1.

Enhanced survival due to thrombolytic therapy

Every trial that has compared thrombolytic therapy with placebo has reached the same conclusion: more patients survive acute MI when they are treated with thrombolytic drugs (Tables 1.1, 1.2). These data are widely believed, and the survival issue is settled. There is no further need, nor would it be ethical, to randomize patients with acute MI to placebo therapy.

It is tempting to compare the percent reduction in mortality from the different trials and to deduce which of the thrombolytic agents is most effective. From Table 1.2, APSAC would appear to "win" with a 50% reduction in mortality. But it is important to recognize that the studies are so different that comparisons are not valid. Look at the different ages, time limitations on therapy, and adjunctive therapeutic combinations (Table 1.1). In addition,

Table 1.1 Mortality trials, all comparing intravenous thrombolytic therapy with placebo

Study*	# Pts	Drug	Time to Rx (hrs)	Age	Adjunctive Rx
GISSI-1	11 806	STK	≤12	No limit	0
ISIS-2	17 187	STK	≤24	No limit	STK — no aspirin STK + aspirin
ISAM	1741	STK	<6	≤75	Heparin, aspirin, warfarin
Western Washington	368	STK	≤6	≤75	Heparin, warfarin
ASSET	5011	rt-PA	≤5	<75	Heparin
AIMS	1258	APSAC	≤6	≤70	Heparin, warfarin, timolol

*Each of these trials is described in Appendix 1.

ECG criteria for entry into the trials was different. ISAM and AIMS required ST segment elevation, GISSI included patients with ST segment depression, and ISIS-2 and ASSET required only "suspected MI." Because of these substantial differences in the protocols, the mortality rates among control (placebo) patients ranged from 7.1 to 13.2% (Table 1.2). For these reasons, determining relative efficacy requires head-to-head comparison of drugs in a single study.

The GISSI-1 trial found that symptomatic reinfarction was twice as common among patients treated with STK when compared with placebo (4% vs 2%). We have heard physicians criticize this result, suggesting that it makes little sense to use a treatment that leaves patients "more unstable after the heart attack." This apparent contradiction is easily explained. Patients treated with thrombolytic therapy who have an open infarct artery are at risk of coronary reocclusion. Most of them have tight and ragged coronary artery plaque with an unstable appearance. The GISSI-1 trial did nothing to "stabilize" the infarct artery; revascularization was seldom applied and use of anticoagulation and/or antianginal therapy was sporadic. Despite the high rate of reinfarction with STK, patients receiving throm-

Table 1.2 Mortality trials, all comparing intravenous thrombolytic therapy with placebo

| Study | Drug | Mortality (%) | | |
		Thrombolytic therapy	Placebo	Difference
GISSI-1	STK	10.7	13.0	18
ISIS-2	STK	9.2	12.0	25
	STK + aspirin	8.0	13.2	42
ISAM	STK	6.3	7.1	11*
Western Washington	STK	6.3	9.6	34*
ASSET	rt-PA	7.2	9.8	26
AIMS	APSAC	6.0	12.0	50

* Not statistically significant. All other trials showed a statistically significant reduction in mortality with thrombolytic therapy (Appendix 1).

bolytic therapy still had an improved survival rate at the time of the 1 year follow-up.

Enhanced LV function after thrombolytic therapy

The most common cause of early, in-hospital death after acute MI is LV failure and not VF. LV failure also identifies the survivors of acute MI who have the highest mortality risk after hospital discharge. In the prethrombolytic era, every study of the natural history of coronary artery disease after MI found that depressed LVEF was the strongest predictor of mortality (Table 1.3).* There have been conclusive studies of STK, rt-PA, and APSAC showing a higher LVEF after thrombolytic therapy than with placebo (Table 1.4).

The LV function issue has importance that transcends its effect on early survival. Most reported studies of survival after throm-

* LVEF is a simple concept. It is the percentage of blood ejected from the left ventricle with each heart beat. From an angiogram (or other imaging study) the volume of the left ventricle can be calculated in both systole and diastole and the simple arithmetic is done. If the volume is 200 ml in diastole and 100 ml in systole, the ejection fraction is 50%. Normal LVEF is usually 50% or higher.

Table 1.3 Influence of LVEF on survival after acute MI (From Taylor, *et al.*, 1980. This study included patients with both Q wave and non-Q wave infarction)

LVEF (%)*	30-month mortality (%)
<30	86
30–39	18
40–49	11
≥50	4

* Cardiac catheterization 12 days after MI.

Table 1.4 LV function in three randomized trials comparing thrombolytic therapy with placebo (see selected reading list)

	STK	rt-PA	APSAC
Number of patients	219	138	231
Time to treatment (hrs)	<4	<4	<5
Mean (hrs)	3.0 ± 0.8	3.2 ± 0.1	3.1 ± 1
Imaging technique	Cath. at 3 weeks	RNA at 10 days	RNA at 19 days
	Global LVEF (%)		
All patients			
Drug treatment	59	53	43
Placebo	53†	46*	39*
Anterior MI			
Drug treatment	57	45	38
Placebo	49*	33*	32*
Inferior MI			
Drug treatment	60	59	47
Placebo	55*	54 ($p = 0.06$)	45 (NS)

* $p < 0.05$
† $p < 0.005$

bolytic therapy reflect a 1-month follow-up (Table 1.2). Knowing that thrombolytic treatment has preserved LV function after MI gives us additional information that has a bearing on long-term survival. Survival with ischemic heart disease is best predicted by LVEF, which is a measurement that reflects cumulative damage to the left ventricle. A patient whose heart attack has been interrupted with thrombolytic therapy will have better preserved LV function, and will be better able to handle a subsequent ischemic event 5 years, 10 years, or 20 years in the future. This insight will not be documented by many studies indicating improved late survival with thrombolytic therapy, as late follow-up is difficult to achieve with large trials. But what we know about LV function and long-term survival with ischemic heart disease leads to the inevitable conclusion that thrombolytic therapy improves long-term prognosis. The goal at each point in the evolution of a patient's illness must be to save as much muscle as possible. A 45-year-old man with acute anterior MI has his best chance to reach age 60 with less myocardial scar and more viable muscle.

The open infarct artery improves survival

Studies of early and late survival after thrombolytic therapy have shown that an open infarct artery conveys a survival benefit independent of demonstrable changes in LV function. Our 6-year survival study of 180 patients who survived hospitalization following Q wave MI and thrombolytic therapy, is the study with the longest follow-up data available. Multivariate analysis of clinical and angiographic variables indicated that three variables were *independent* predictors of death at 6 years:
1 diabetes;
2 anterior location of MI; and
3 a closed infarct artery at catheterization within 24 hours of thrombolytic therapy.

Anterior location of MI is a reliable marker of low ejection fraction in patients with Q wave MI. The lowest-risk group of patients, those with inferior MI, had a higher survival rate with an open infarct artery. Similarly, the highest-risk patients with anterior MI also had improved 6-year survival if they had an open infarct artery following thrombolytic therapy. The highest-risk patients with a combination of diabetes, anterior infarction, and a closed infarct artery had 75% 6-year mortality rate compared with a 33% mortality rate for similar patients with an open infarct artery (Fig. 1.1). Other studies support this finding that patients who have successful thrombolysis fare better than patients who fail to open the infarct artery with thrombolytic treatment. LV function remains an important determinant of survival, but an open artery provides additional benefit.

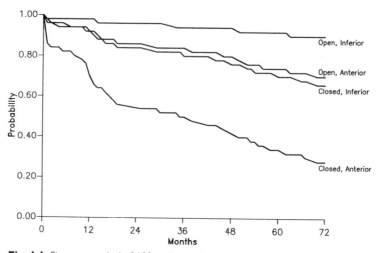

Fig. 1.1 Six-year survival of 180 patients who were treated with thrombolytic agents and survived initial hospitalization. Multivariate analysis showed that diabetes, anterior location of MI, and a closed infarct artery at catheterization early after MI were independent predictors of death. This figure describes highest-risk patients with diabetes, and demonstrates the independence of infarct location and status of the infarct artery as predictors of mortality. An open infarct artery within 24 hours of thrombolytic therapy favorably influenced survival both in lower-risk patients with inferior MI as well as higher-risk patients with anterior MI. In this study, an open infarct artery also favorably influenced survival independent of predischarge LVEF.

It is not clear why an open infarct artery is beneficial independent of LV function. The open artery may be a better source for collateral flow to other, stenosed coronary arteries. Continued flow in the infarct zone may reduce the potential for cardiac arrhythmia. The beneficial effect may be related to improved contractility in both the infarct and peri-infarction zones that is not currently measurable using state-of-the-art, yet gross techniques such as angiography, echocardiography, or RNA. As is often observed during surgery, most patients after thrombolytic therapy appear to have islets of viable muscle, and these remnants of viable muscle may be better preserved with an open artery. While small amounts of muscle may not affect gross measurements of LV function, they may be enough to prevent alterations of LV geometry including infarct expansion and aneurysm formation.

Morbidity is reduced by thrombolytic therapy

Placebo-controlled trials have shown a lower incidence of heart failure among patients treated with thrombolytic therapy. This is consistent with the finding of better preserved LV function after thrombolysis (Table 1.4). A benign clinical course may follow thrombolytic therapy. The patients have better exercise tolerance, less fatigue, and fewer serious late arrhythmias, all effects of better LV function. Their hospitalization time is shortened, and this reduces the cost of care.

The most frustrating patients we care for are those with end-stage LV failure. We used to observe large numbers of young patients, usually men, with ischemic cardiomyopathy and severe disability. Sudden death was common. While alive they were unable to work, had little vigor, spent excessive time in the doctor's office, and were miserable.

In central Illinois, with widespread application of thrombolytic therapy over the last decade, it is less common for us to see patients with ischemic cardiomyopathy. Patients treated with thrombolytic therapy have a better chance of recovering after their MI with a high level of functional ability.

Do I have to use thrombolytic therapy?

As far as we are concerned, you do if you propose to care for patients with acute MI. A recent survey of physicians who routinely see patients with acute MI found that cardiologists were three times as likely to use thrombolytic drugs as family practitioners and twice as likely as internists. The drug companies selling thrombolytic agents tell us that competing for market share with other drugs is not their main problem. Instead, they are frustrated by the small percentage of patients with MI receiving any thrombolytic agent. Data proving efficacy are too compelling. You cannot afford to care for patients with acute MI unless you can appropriately apply thrombolytic therapy.

The good news is that you *can* do it and do it well. In our central Illinois experience we compared patients who were treated in community hospitals by primary care physicians with patients treated in the tertiary referral center, usually by a cardiologist (Table 1.5). The results clearly demonstrated that the community hospital patients did as well as those treated in the referral center, and they were treated as early. Hospital survival was as good.

Table 1.5 Thrombolytic therapy in the community hospital vs referral center — the central Illinois experience (1982–87) with intravenous STK in 1012 patients (From Taylor, et al., 1990)

	Community hospital	Referral center
Number pts	816	196
Age	56 ± 11	57 ± 11
Infarct Location		
Anterior	340 (42%)	70 (36%)
Inferior	465 (57%)	122 (62%)
Time to Rx (min)	173 ± 96	161 ± 76
Open infarct artery*	710 (87%)	162 (83%)
LVEF†	49 ± 14%	51 ± 14%
Death in hospital	39 (5%)	12 (6%)
Complications		
Stroke	2 (0.3%)	1 (0.5%)
Any bleed	82 (10.1%)	26 (13.3%)
Bleed→transfusion	17 (2.1%)	7 (3.6%)

* At catheterization ≤ 2 days after thrombolytic therapy. Community hospital patients were transferred for cardiac catheterization.
† LVEF, before hospital discharge. An RNA was performed in 62% of patients in the community hospital group and 67% in the referral center group.

Table 1.6 Follow-up mortality study of 192 patients treated with STK in 1981–83 (From Taylor, et al., 1989)

	Community hospital	Referral center
Initial hospitalization	8/113 (7%)	4/79 (5%)
Follow-up		
20-month	5/105 (4.8%)	2/75 (3%)
6-year	5/100 (5%)	9/73 (12%)
Cumulative		
20-month	13/113 (12%)	6/79 (8%)
6-year	18/113 (16%)	15/79 (19%)

Complication rates were no higher. Our follow-up studies in the subset treated before 1984 have shown that 20-month and 6-year survivals were equal or better for patients treated in community hospitals (Table 1.6).

We have had the opportunity to work closely with doctors in these community hospitals who, in a real sense, have pioneered thrombolytic therapy at the grass roots level. We now know that any doctor who has experience caring for patients with acute MI, and who is able to use heparin, will be able to use thrombolytic drugs. It is not that hard, and the benefits are manifest.

Selected reading

Gersh BJ. Benefits of the open artery: Beyond myocardial salvage. J Myocardial Ischemia 1990;2:15–37.

Hlatky MA, Cotugno H, O'Connor C, Mark DB, Prior DB, Califf RM. Adoption of thrombolytic therapy in the management of acute myocardial infarction. Am J Cardiol 1988;61:510–4.

Schroder R. A review of thrombolysis mortality trials: ISAM to ASSET. J Interven Cardiol 1990;3:139–44.

Stone PH, Muller JE, Hartwell T, et al. The effect of diabetes mellitus on prognosis and serial left ventricular function after acute myocardial infarction: Contribution of both coronary disease and diastolic left ventricular dysfunction to the adverse prognosis. J Am Coll Cardiol 1989;14:49–57.

Sutton JM, Taylor GJ, Mikell FL, et al. Thrombolytic therapy followed by early revascularization for acute myocardial infarction. Am J Cardiol 1986;57:1227–31.

Taylor GJ, Song A, Moses HW, et al. The primary care physician and thrombolytic therapy for acute myocardial infarction: Comparison of intravenous streptokinase in community hospitals and the tertiary referral center. J Am Board Fam Pract 1990;3:1–6.

Taylor GJ, Song A, Korsmeyer C, et al. Six year survival after thrombolysis for acute myocardial infarction. Circulation 1989;80(Suppl):11–520.

Taylor GJ, Humphries O, Mellits ED, et al. Predictors of clinical course, coronary anatomy and left ventricular function after recovery from acute myocardial infarction. Circulation 1980;62:960–70.

LV function studies

Bassand JP, Machecourt J, Cassagnes J, et al. Multicenter trial of intravenous anisoylated plasminogen streptokinase activator complex (APSAC) in acute myocardial infarction: Effects on infarct size and left ventricular function. J Am Coll Cardiol 1989;13:988–97.

Guerci AD, Gerstenblith G, Brinker JA, et al. A randomized trial of intravenous tissue plasminogen activator for acute myocardial infarction with subsequent randomization to elective coronary angioplasty. N Engl J Med 1987;317:1613–18.

White HD, Norris RM, Brown MA, et al. Effect of intravenous streptokinase on left ventricular function and early survival after acute myocardial infarction. N Engl J Med 1987;317:850–55.

Survival studies

AIMS Trial Study Group. Effect of intravenous APSAC on mortality after acute myocardial infarction: Preliminary report of a placebo-controlled clinical trial. Lancet 1988;1:545–49.

GISSI. Effectiveness of thrombolytic treatment in acute myocardial infarction. Lancet 1986;1:397–402.

ISAM Study Group. A prospective trial of intravenous streptokinase in acute myocardial infarction (ISAM): Mortality, morbidity and infarct size at 21 days. N Engl J Med 1986;324:1465–71.

ISIS-2 Collaborative Group. Randomized trial of intravenous streptokinase, oral aspirin, both, or neither among 17187 cases of suspected acute myocardial infarction: ISIS-2*. J Am Coll Cardiol 1988;12: 3–13A.

Kennedy JW, Martim GV, Davis KB, et al. The Western Washington intravenous streptokinase in acute myocardial infarction randomized trial. Circulation 1988;77:345–52.

Wilcox RG, Von der Lippe G, Olsson CG, et al. Trial of tissue plasminogen activator for mortality reduction in acute myocardial infarction. Anglo-Scandinavian study of early thrombolysis (ASSET). Lancet 1988;2:525–30.

Chapter 2

Diagnosis of acute MI; clinical and electrocardiographic findings

Chapters 2 and 3 are basic and brief reviews focusing on diagnostic and patient selection issues that allow you to use thrombolytic therapy for the right patient with acute MI, and to avoid it when it is less beneficial or excessively risky. For 80% of patients with chest pain the proper clinical decision is obvious. What that means, unfortunately, is that you will commonly face a patient with either borderline or uncertain indications for thrombolytic therapy. We often find this the case when we, as cardiologists, are evaluating patients with chest pain. What we recommend to you, and what we do ourselves when the decision is tough, is get a consultation. We call a colleague for another opinion. Discussing the case often helps us to understand the clinical issues more clearly, and a colleague frequently thinks of something that makes the treatment decision obvious. It is important to document this in the medical record. These are sick patients and not every treatment will be successful, but your description of your thought process and the thoughts of a consultant on the chart will document that you have done your best. It is as important to state your reasons for avoiding thrombolytic therapy as it is to outline reasons to treat. If you work in an emergency department and see patients with acute MI you need the telephone numbers of suitable consultants.

Those who have worked in the CCU and who are comfortable with ECG interpretation may find this review simplistic, but those of you who work in an emergency department may have less experience evaluating patients with chest pain or training in ECG interpretation. Much of this chapter describes our approach to patient evaluation and ECG interpretation.

Clinical presentation

Acute coronary thrombosis or occlusion produces immediate symptoms. When balloon catheters are inflated in coronary arte-

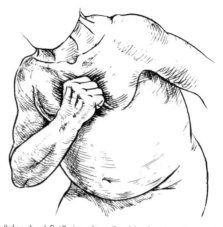

Fig. 2.1 The "clenched fist" sign described by Levine. A surprising percentage of patients describe severe ischemic pain in this fashion, and it is a fair indicator that the pain is cardiac. Ischemic pain is midchest in location. When a patient points to a spot on the left side and states that "it hurts over my heart," it probably is noncardiac. A problem with a history, of course, is that location and quality of pain are so variable among patients.

ries producing total occlusion, pain usually develops within a minute. Angina is a midchest, retrosternal pain. With a heart attack the pain is also retrosternal but may occupy most of the chest. Patients often describe it as heavy, squeezing, crushing, band-like, burning, aching pain. Often they will illustrate their pain with a fist clenched over midchest; the "fist sign" or "Levine sign" (Fig. 2.1). When a patient points to the left side with one finger and says, "It hurts over may heart," it is less likely to be cardiac. While the pain of angina pectoris may be mild (many patients say it is "not a pain"), the pain of MI, while qualitatively similar, usually is severe.

Most patients with MI have associated symptoms including shortness of breath, cold sweat, or nausea. But there are also patients who come in with mild and/or atypical pain involving an arm, a wrist, the jaw, with "weakness," or with no symptoms at all. An atypical presentation is more likely in older patients, women, and those with diabetes. In the emergency department you are dealing with patients who have symptoms at least sufficiently severe to cause them to seek medical care. Acute MI may be precipitated by heavy physical activity such as shoveling snow. Just as often it occurs at rest or during sleep. More than half the

Table 2.1 Differential diagnosis of acute chest pain

MI
Pericarditis
Dissecting aortic aneurysm
Dissecting aneurysm with occlusion of a coronary artery and MI
Pulmonary hypertension
Myocarditis
Pleurisy
Pneumothorax
Pulmonary embolus
Costochondritis (Tietze's syndrome)
Bursitis
Thoracic outlet syndrome
Herpes zoster
Cervical arthritis/radiculitis
Peptic esophagitis
Peptic ulcer
Esophageal rupture
Hiatus hernia
Pylorospasm
Gallbladder disease
Splenic flexure syndrome
Psychogenic chest pain
And others

patients will give a history of having some mild discomfort in the weeks before a heart attack. Often this was perceived as indigestion, arthritis, etc.

It is important to accurately record the time of onset of chest pain. The duration of pain before arrival at the hospital and thrombolytic therapy have bearing on prognosis. Precise identification of onset of symptoms is difficult for many patients. Some of them have had symptoms that waxed and waned during the day or two before MI. The onset of acute MI is usually different from these premonitory symptoms. Either it is more severe or it doesn't go away. That change in symptoms identifies the onset of infarction.

The differential diagnosis of chest pain is lengthy (Table 2.1). Many of these conditions can be excluded with a history and physical examination. As with any illness, obtaining accurate history is the clinician's first job. But you should not waste time. This should be a directed history aimed both at establishing a clinical diagnosis and excluding contraindications to thrombolytic

Table 2.2 Killip classification (From Killip and Kimball's (1967) description of 250 patients with acute MI treated in 1965−66)

Class	Clinical findings	Hospital mortality (%)
I	No evidence for CHF	6
II	CHF (Rales, S₃ gallop, JVD)	17
III	Pulmonary edema	38
IV	Cardiogenic shock	81

JVD, jugular venous distension. Cardiogenic shock was defined as systolic blood pressure ≤90 mmHg plus oliguria and often obtundation.

therapy. Get a clear description of the pain. Do a systems review of possible illnesses that increase bleeding risk. After treating a patient who had bumped his head before admission and who had an intracerebral bleed after STK treatment, we now routinely examine patients for signs of head trauma. During acute MI, patients and families commonly forget what they consider to be minor events. A small contusion can turn into a monstrous hematoma following thrombolytic therapy.

The absence of any risk factors for coronary heart disease is unusual in patients with acute MI. Patients with diabetes are more likely to have atypical symptoms or perhaps no symptoms at all. A recent patient with diabetic ketoacidosis was found to have acute MI on the admission ECG. Her painless infarction precipitated ketoacidosis.

A history of poorly-controlled hypertension may be important, as such patients are at higher risk for intracranial bleeding. A prior history of transient ischemic attack (TIA) or stroke may also increase the risk of intracranial bleeding.

On examination, a patient with acute MI appears ill and anxious. The skin is cold and clammy. Examine the chest and jugular veins for evidence of heart failure. As S₄ gallop is common. If there is papillary muscle ischemia there may be a soft systolic murmur (mitral regurgitation). But these physical findings are nonspecific. There are no cardiac findings that point directly to the diagnosis of acute MI.

While physical examination adds little to the diagnosis of MI, it may help in establishing mortality risk of the MI. Table 2.2 outlines the Killip classification. While the mortality rates observed by Killip and Kimball in 1967 have been altered by thrombolytic therapy, it is still true that patients with CHF, and especially Killip class III or IV, have the worst prognosis. The Killip classification therefore becomes an important element in weighing risk vs benefits of thrombolytic therapy for the individual patient.

The ECG

We are most confident making a diagnosis of acute MI using the triad of:
1 chest pain;
2 typical ECG changes;
3 abnormalities in cardiac enzymes indicating leakage of the injured cells' contents into the blood stream.

CK may not rise until 12 hours after the onset of MI. The cardiac enzymes therefore play no role in deciding to use thrombolytic agents when evaluating a patient with recent onset of pain.

The decision to treat with thrombolytic therapy boils down to history and the ECG. For practical purposes, this is all you need and all that you have available.

If the initial ECG does not indicate acute MI, look carefully for another etiology of chest pain (Table 2.1). On the other hand, it may be important to repeat the ECG in 15–30 minutes. We are amazed how often the second or even third ECG shows dramatic and diagnostic changes of acute MI when the first one did not. Figures 2.2(A) and 2.2(B) are a pair of ECGs from a patient who had chest pain suggesting MI. There was minimal ST segment elevation in inferior leads, nothing overwhelming. A repeat ECG 25 minutes later was far more impressive with ST segment elevation indicating a need for thrombolytic therapy.

Basic ECG interpretation

The ECG is a volt meter. When heart muscle is depolarized, an electrical field is generated that can be detected at the surface of the body using a sensitive volt meter. Figure 2.3 is a schematic of the typical ECG pattern. The cardiac cycle begins with spontaneous depolarization of the sinoatrial (SA) node, the normal "pacemaker" of the heart. The SA node fires automatically at 60–100 beats/minute, and this rate of firing is influenced by the autonomic nervous system. It slows with stimulation of the vagus nerve (parasympathetic activation), and it increases under the influence of catacholamines (sympathetic activation). Depolariza-

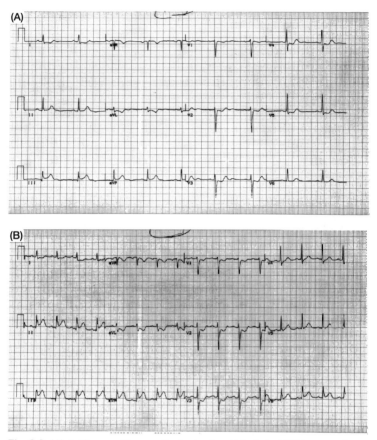

Fig. 2.2 (A) A 42-year-old man with chest pain which started 1½ hours earlier. This ECG shows minimal ST segment elevation in leads III and aVF, but the changes are small enough that there is uncertainty. (B) A repeat ECG 25 minutes later as his pain intensified showed marked ST segment elevation in inferior leads as well as reciprocal ST segment depression in anterolateral leads. Thrombolytic therapy clearly is indicated for acute inferior infarction.

tion of the SA node does not produce a measurable current, but the subsequent depolarization of both left and right atria generates the current that is the P wave on the surface ECG.

There is a layer of insulation between the atria and the ventricles preventing direct passage of current between them. Instead, current is funneled through the atrioventricular (AV) node. Conduction in the AV node is slower than in other cardiac tissue. This delay of conduction in the AV node, the PR interval on the

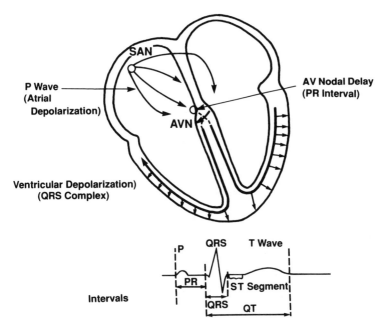

Fig. 2.3 The SA node, located in the high right atrium, is the cardiac "pacemaker." It fires at a rate of 60–100 beats/minute and is influenced by both sympathetic and parasympathetic tone. Atrial muscle depolarization produces enough current to cause a deflection, the P wave, on the surface ECG. The wave of depolarization is funneled into the AV node, located at the junction of the atrial and ventricular septa. Current is delayed in the AV node producing the PR interval. This delay allows time for atrial contraction which completes the filling of the ventricles. Current exits the AV node into the common bundle of His and shortly divides into the left and right bundle branches. Initial depolarization of the interventricular septum takes place from the left to right side. Current then moves through the left and right bundle branches into the ventricular myocardium producing the QRS complex. The left ventricle is much thicker than the right and thus generates more voltage. LV depolarization therefore dominates the QRS complex. The ventricle is repolarized producing the T wave on the ECG. No voltage is apparent between the end of the QRS and the T wave. This ST segment shifts up (ST segment elevation) or down (ST segment depression) with varying degrees of ischemia.

ECG, allows time for atrial contraction before the ventricles are activated and contract.

Current exits the AV node, passes through the common bundle of His, then simultaneously through left and right bundles into the Purkinje system, and then to the ventricular myocardium. Depolarization of the much thicker ventricular myocardium pro-

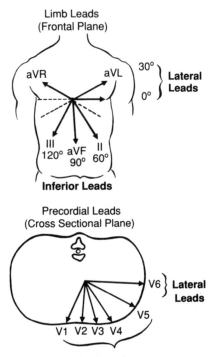

Fig. 2.4 Spatial orientation of ECG leads. Each of the ECG leads functions as a volt meter and has spatial orientation (as voltage is a vector). The limb leads (I, II, III, aVR, aVL, aVF) sense voltage generated by the heart in the frontal plane. The precordial leads (V1–V6) sense voltage in the cross-sectional plane. As an example, lead AVF records voltage moving directly downward, 90° from horizontal. Leads which have an inferior orientation (II, III, aVF) sensitively detect changes from the inferior surface of the heart. Anterior precordial leads are most sensitive in detecting anterior wall changes. Leads with lateral orientation (I, aVL, V6) best detect lateral wall changes.

duces the largest deflection on the surface ECG, the QRS complex. The ventricular myocardium is then repolarized, and this produces the T wave.

In a sense, each ECG lead is a separate volt meter which examines electrical forces moving through the heart in a specific spatial orientation (Fig. 2.4). The inferior leads are most sensitive to electrical forces moving toward the inferior surface of the heart. Ischemia of the inferior wall thus produces the greatest changes in these inferior leads (II, III, and aVF). Anterior myocardial changes are best detected by leads overlying the anterior

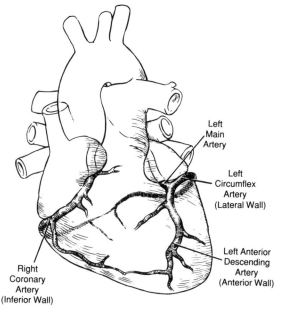

Fig. 2.5 There are three major coronary branches. The right coronary artery supplies the inferior surface of the heart; occlusion causes changes in "inferior leads" (II, III, aVF). The anterior descending artery supplies the majority of anterior wall muscle as well as much of the interventricular septum, and occlusion causes changes in anterior precordial leads. The circumflex artery wraps around the lateral wall and is most likely to cause changes in the lateral leads.

In the figure, the following labels appear: Left Main Artery; Left Circumflex Artery (Lateral Wall); Left Anterior Descending Artery (Anterior Wall); Right Coronary Artery (Inferior Wall).

wall of the heart (precordial leads V1–V5). Lateral wall changes are best seen in left lateral leads (I, aVL, and V6).

Likewise, the "location" of ECG changes roughly predicts the coronary artery responsible for the ischemic syndrome (Fig. 2.5). Eighty-five percent of patients who have changes in leads II, III, and aVF (inferior leads) have obstruction of the right coronary artery which supplies the inferior surface of the heart. Anterior (V1–V5) changes generally indicate obstruction of the left anterior descending artery. Lateral changes (I, aVL, or V6) indicate circumflex artery (or diagonal branch) obstruction.

When changes affect both anterior and lateral leads, (V1–V6, I, aVL) the MI is considered "anterolateral." Changes in inferior and lateral leads (II, III, aVF, I, aVL, V6), are "inferolateral." More diffuse ECG changes do not indicate simultaneous occlusion of two vessels to two vascular distributions. Instead, patients with anterolateral MI have occlusion of an anterior descending artery

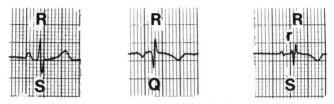

Fig. 2.6 QRS nomenclature. Any positive deflection is an R wave. An initial negative deflection is referred to as a Q wave. A negative deflection following an R wave is an S wave. Small, low-voltage deflections may be designated with lower case letters.

with branches to the lateral wall. A patient with inferolateral MI usually has occlusion of a right coronary artery with a large distal branch wrapping around to the lateral wall. These infarcts, with changes seen more broadly in more ECG leads, are larger because of occlusion of bigger arteries supplying more muscle.

The Q, R, and S waves are produced by ventricular muscle depolarization. If the initial deflection is negative it is called a Q wave (Fig. 2.6). If the initial wave or any subsequent wave is positive it is called an R wave. A negative wave following an R wave is called an S wave. The amplitude of deflection does not change this nomenclature, although low voltage deflections may be labeled with lower case letters, (i.e. rSR).

Ischemic patterns on the ECG

Myocardial ischemia and injury produce changes in the QRS complex, the ST segment, or the T wave (Fig. 2.7). Animal studies using ECGs recorded from the surface of the heart have shown that Q waves indicate full thickness, "transmural" injury, or scar tissue. Various patterns of ST and T wave changes indicate different degrees of ischemia and/or acute injury. In addition to animal laboratory data, coronary angiography during acute ischemic syndromes has allowed us to correlate ECG changes to the status of the coronary artery and to LV contraction patterns.

The ECG pattern that is most specific and diagnostic for myocardial scar is the Q wave (Fig. 2.7). But Q waves may appear late in the course of acute MI, often when injury is complete. For purposes of rapid diagnosis of acute MI, the ECG patterns of early infarction are much more important, as they are the basis for deciding to use thrombolytic therapy. Here are the ECG patterns commonly encountered in patients with acute chest pain.

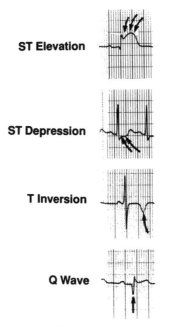

ST Elevation

ST Depression

T Inversion

Q Wave

Fig. 2.7 ECG patterns that may indicate acute ischemia or ischemic injury. ST segment elevation is the one to look for; this usually indicates transmural ischemia and is the earliest ECG manifestation of the "Q-wave" MI. The size of the MI is roughly proportional to the number of leads with ST segment elevation. ST segment depression is a nonspecific finding; when associated with chest pain and when it is new when compared with earlier tracings, it means ischemia. This is what a positive stress ECG looks like. T wave inversion also may be a nonspecific finding; when it is new it may mean nontransmural ischemia and is the typical ECG pattern of non-Q wave MI. The Q wave indicates transmural injury; Q waves in more ECG leads generally mean a large MI. An isolated Q wave in just V1 or lead III may be normal.

ST segment elevation and chest pain

The "ST segment elevation MI" is an unequivocal indication for thrombolytic therapy (Fig. 2.7). Patients who have ST segment elevation in early infarction usually progress to Q wave formation and have full–thickness or "transmural" injury of the left ventricle. The currently accepted nomenclature is "Q wave" rather than "transmural" MI. Since Q waves are not present at the time of initial presentation with acute MI, we will refer to "ST segment elevation MI."

Emergency angiography in patients with ST segment elevation and ischemic chest pain almost always shows occlusion of the

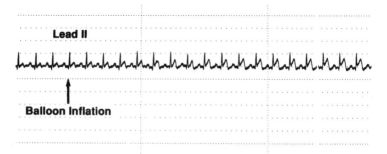

Fig. 2.8 During balloon dilatation of the right coronary artery, the occluded balloon blocked flow causing total ischemia. This continuous tracing shows that ST segment elevation in lead II developed promptly, within 30 seconds of occlusion of the artery.

coronary artery. When we occlude coronary arteries in the catheterization laboratory during balloon dilatation, the usual response is ST segment elevation, and it develops rapidly, within 1 minute (Fig. 2.8). Chest pain also appears promptly, and contractility of the ischemic region is dramatically depressed within 5–15 heart beats.

Patients with ST segment elevation in the anterior (V leads) are having acute anterior infarction. The 54-year-old patient with the ECG in Figure 2.9 arrived 30 minutes after onset of pain, and his ECG showed minimal ST segment elevation in leads V3–V6. A repeat ECG 20 minutes later indicated large anterolateral infarction with ST segment elevation in V2–V6. The next day he had developed (or "evolved") Q waves; CK rose to 3250 iu. Before discharge, coronary angiography showed occlusion of the anterior descending artery and a LVEF of 22%.* He never returned to work and currently takes four cardiac medications. He sees his doctor twice a month to adjust his diuretic dose. Unfortunately, he had his anterior MI a month before his hospital started a program of thrombolytic therapy.

Acute inferior infarction causes ST segment elevation in the "inferior" leads II, III, and aVF (Figs 2.4, 2.5). The 52-year-old

---

* Normal LVEF is above 50%. Patients with ejection fraction 30–40% still have fair exercise tolerance. Below 25%, most have exercise limitations. The Social Security Administration uses an ejection fraction of 30% or less as the criterion for disability benefits with heart failure.

woman with the ECG in Figure 2.10(A) had ST segment elevation in the inferior leads. She also had ST segment elevation
in lateral leads indicating more widespread, "inferolateral"
ischemia. In addition to ST segment elevation there was ST segment depression in the anterior leads. Q waves were apparent the
next day (Fig. 2.10B).

This "reciprocal" ST segment depression with inferior MI was
initially attributed to clinically unimportant electrical phenomena.
In the last decade we have learned that patients with inferior MI
who have anterior and/or lateral reciprocal ST segment depres-

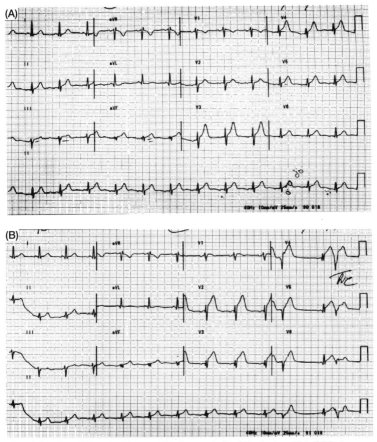

Fig. 2.9 (A) A 54-year-old man with chest pain for 30 minutes. This ECG shows
minimal, but suspicious ST segment elevation in anterior leads. (B) The ECG was
repeated 20 minutes later. This tracing shows marked ST segment elevation in
anterior and lateral leads. Treat with thrombolytic therapy.

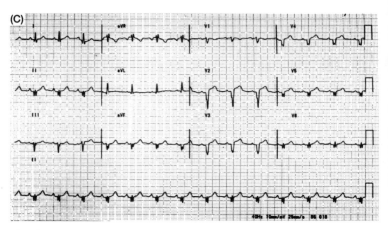

Fig. 2.9 (C) The next morning a repeat ECG showed development of Q waves in leads V1–V6, roughly the same leads which had ST segment elevation. He also had left anterior fascicular block (marked left axis deviation and ventricular conduction delay).

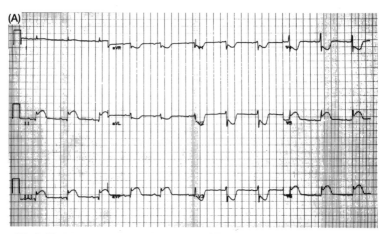

Fig. 2.10 (A) Acute inferior infarction with ST segment elevation in leads II, III, and aVF. This appears to be a large MI as there is also ST segment elevation in leads V5–V6 suggesting involvement of the lateral wall, a combination often referred to as "inferolateral" ischemia. This patient also has reciprocal ST segment depression in the anterior leads as well as aVL.

sion are having more widespread ischemia. They have greater CK release and at the time of hospital discharge, have lower LVEF. They have larger heart attacks because they have a right coronary artery that supplies not only the inferior wall but a portion of the

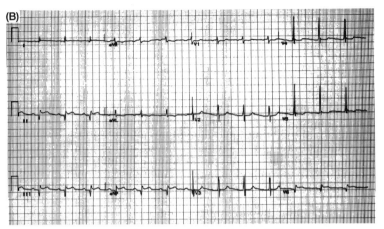

Fig. 2.10 (B) The next day Q waves had evolved in leads II, III, aVF and there is still mild ST segment elevation in the inferior leads. Lateral and anterior ST wave changes have resolved.

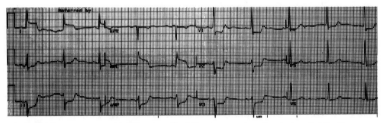

Fig. 2.11 Acute lateral infarction with ST segment elevation in I and aVL. Our experience is that most patients with circumflex artery occlusion and acute lateral MI do not have ST segment elevation; the lateral wall seems to be an electrocardiographically "silent" area of the heart.

lateral wall or apex as well (producing the ST segment changes in the anterior and/or lateral leads). In our earlier studies of thrombolytic therapy we limited treatment to patients with inferior MI who also had reciprocal ST segment depression in the anterior or lateral leads in an effort to treat only large inferior MIs. Now we treat all patients with inferior MI, but are especially concerned about those who have reciprocal ST segment depression. A more thorough discussion of patient selection issues is found in Chapter 3.

ST segment elevation in I, aVL, and lateral precordial leads (V5–V6), indicates acute lateral infarction (Fig. 2.11). This usually follows occlusion of the circumflex artery or a diagonal

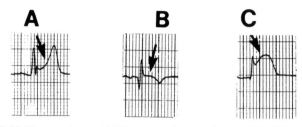

Fig. 2.12 Three patients with ST segment elevation. Patient A has ST segment elevation but maintains the normal, upward concavity of the ST segment. This pattern of ST segment elevation may mean ischemia, but it could also be caused by other conditions (pericarditis, early repolarization, etc.). Patient B has lost some of the upward concavity and has a "flat" ST segment. In addition, this patient has a small Q wave and biphasic T waves; the diagnosis of ischemia is fairly certain. Patient C has marked ST segment elevation with upwardly convex ST segments. This is the more typical pattern of acute, transmural ischemia.

branch of the anterior descending artery (Fig. 2.5). As noted above, an occasional patient with a large right coronary artery with branches to the low lateral wall as well as to the inferior wall will have lateral ST segment elevation during acute inferior MI (Fig. 2.10A). This inferolateral infarct pattern indicates an unusually large MI, as the number of leads with ST segment elevation is roughly proportional to the extent of ischemic injury.

The size of the MI is roughly proportional to the number of ECG leads with ischemic ST segment elevation. This is true with any MI. You can estimate the size of the MI by simply counting the number of leads with ST segment elevation (a formula to convert this to gram-equivalent of heart muscle is provided by Aldrich, *et al.*, 1988).

The shape of the ST segments may help with diagnosis. Normally the ST segment is upwardly concave (Fig. 2.12). But with transmural ischemia and ST segment elevation, the ST segment may flatten or become upwardly convex. This feature is useful in differentiating the ST segment elevation of ischemia from that seen with pericarditis or with early repolarization (Chapter 3).

Chest pain with BBB

We excluded patients with left BBB from our early trials as the conduction abnormality may obscure the diagnosis of acute MI. We wished to study a pure population. The large ISIS-2 and GISSI-1 trials, both comparing thrombolytic agents to placebo, included patients with acute chest pain and BBB. Both studies found that patients with clinical MI (typical chest pain) and BBB had improved survival with thrombolytic therapy. One reason for this is the high mortality rate seen with BBB and acute MI, as BBB may indicate a large acute infarction or pre-existing LV dysfunction. The combination of chest pain typical for acute MI and BBB is now an accepted indication for thrombolytic therapy.

BBB is the interruption of nerve conduction through either the left or right bundles, the system of nerves moving through the interventricular septum (Fig. 2.3). Block of conduction in either the left or right bundle delays passage of current to the ventricle and thus causes broadening of the QRS complex. (The "x axis" of the ECG is time, each small square = 0.04 seconds). Normally, QRS duration is less than 0.12 seconds (Fig. 2.3). BBB causes broadening of the QRS complex beyond 0.12 seconds.

Right BBB

When the right bundle branch is blocked, initial depolarization of the interventricular septum is not affected (Fig. 2.13). For this reason, the initial portion of the QRS is not changed. But the end of the QRS is slurred since depolarization of the right side of the heart is delayed. In a sense, there is terminal conduction delay with the terminal (tail-end) electrical forces oriented anteriorly and to the right, the last region to be activated. This produces an rSR pattern in lead V1. When the right bundle is blocked, the right side is the last area of the ventricles to be depolarized, and thus terminal forces in right sided leads (V1) are positive. (When current is moving toward a lead it produces a positive deflection in the QRS complex; when current is moving away from the lead it produces a negative deflection.) The terminal QRS forces in left-sided leads (I, aVL, V6) would be negative as current is moving away from them and toward the right side.

The bulk of the left ventricle (including the septum) is activated normally in patients with right BBB. You may therefore expect to see the usual MI patterns with ST segment elevation and subsequent development of Q waves. Thus, with right BBB you will be able to diagnose MI from the initial ECG.

Figure 2.14 presents ECGs from two patients with right BBB having acute MI. Both ST segment changes and Q waves can be reliably interpreted despite the presence of right BBB. You can rely on usual ECG patterns of infarction.

Recent information indicates that patients who have anterior

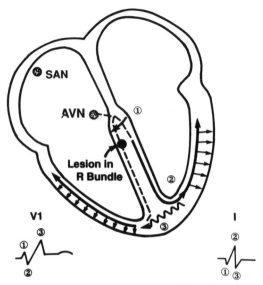

Fig. 2.13 Sequence of ventricular activation in right BBB with representative tracings from leads I and V1. (1) Initial left to right depolarization of the septum (the normal sequence) produces a positive deflection (r wave) in V1. (2) Because the right bundle is blocked, the left bundle branch and left ventricle are activated next, and this produces the S wave in V1. (3) The wave of depolarization passes from the left side over to the right side so that RV depolarization occurs at the end of the QRS complex and produces the terminal R wave in V1. The reverse is seen in lead I in this example. The keys to the diagnosis of right BBB are a wide QRS complex, rSR pattern in V1, and terminal forces to the right (V1).

MI and right BBB have a much higher mortality rate than those with normal conduction. Right BBB may indicate that more myocardium is ischemic, with injury including the interventricular septum. Anatomically, it may indicate that the anterior descending artery is blocked proximally, affecting more of the septal perforating branches. For this reason, acute infarction and especially anterior MI with right BBB are powerful indicators for thrombolytic therapy.

Left BBB (Fig. 2.15)
This conduction abnormality distorts the entire QRS complex and makes diagnosis of acute MI difficult. Patients with left BBB have initial depolarization of the right side of the heart with late depolarization of the left side. In addition to a widened QRS complex, terminal QRS forces are pointed to the left, towards

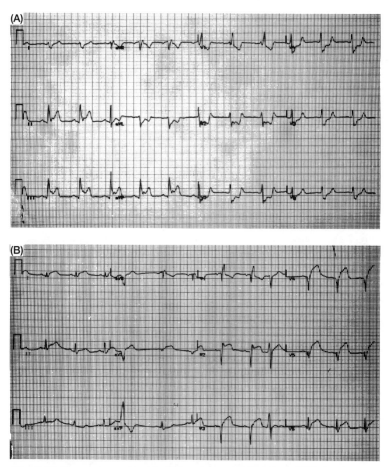

Fig. 2.14 Two patients with right BBB and acute MI. Both have QRS duration greater than 0.12 seconds and rSR pattern in V1. Patient (A) has ST segment elevation in inferior leads with reciprocal ST segment depression in V2–V5 and aVL indicating large inferior MI. Patient (B) has ST segment elevation in V2–V6 as well as Q waves indicating anterior MI. The diagnosis of acute MI is not changed by the presence of right BBB.

leads I, aVL, and V6 (Fig. 2.15). There is little voltage generated by depolarization of the thin-walled right ventricle, and little negative deflection is seen in these left-sided leads. Left BBB may also cause shifts in ST segments and T waves (Fig. 2.16), and these ST segment changes do not necessarily indicate active ischemia. If there is a big change in the ST segments or T waves

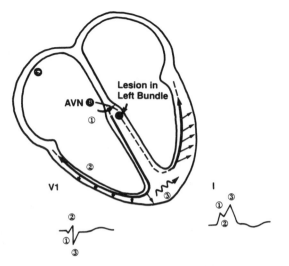

Fig. 2.15 Sequence of ventricular activation in left BBB. After current passes through the AV node, (1) normal left to right depolarization of the septum is interrupted by the blocked left bundle. The septum thus depolarizes from right to left. This produces an initially positive deflection in left-sided leads, V6 and aVL. (2) Next, the right bundle activates the right ventricle, but this produces little current as the right ventricle is thin–walled. A small positive deflection may be seen in lead V1 or a negative "glitch" in lead I. (3) Current moves from the right side across to the left with late depolarization of the thick-walled left ventricle which produces the highest voltage deflection. The keys to diagnosis of left BBB are wide QRS complex, loss of the initial negative deflection in left-sided leads, and terminal QRS forces toward the left side (I, aVL, V6).

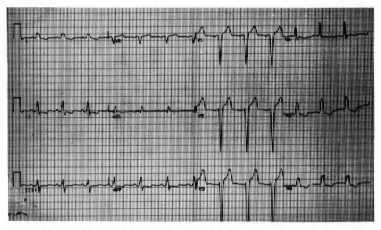

Fig. 2.16 A patient with left BBB. There is ST segment elevation in leads V1–V3 as well as down-sloping ST segments with depression in inferior and lateral leads. But this patient had no chest pain and was not having acute MI. ST segment changes and Q waves are not reliable indicators of MI in the presence of left BBB.

when compared with previous ECGs, acute ischemia may be inferred. Usually the clinician must make a decision about thrombolytic therapy based on clinical symptoms.

New left BBB (when compared with an old ECG) and acute infarction indicates an unusually large amount of injury and a high mortality risk. Urgent thrombolysis is needed. The patient may need a temporary pacemaker. His or her family should be aware that prognosis is poor. Even more so than right BBB, this indicates an especially large area of myocardium that is ischemic.

Q waves and chest pain

Q waves take hours to develop. If the patient presents with chest pain and already has Q waves, is it too late to give thrombolytic therapy? The Q waves could mean a prior MI. If so, the patient has an especially high mortality risk and should be treated. When the Q waves are related to the present infarction, it may mean an earlier onset of MI than indicated by the history. Another possibility is early reperfusion, which can accelerate development of Q waves. The patient may then have reocclusion of the coronary artery with return of pain and ST segment elevation.

The persistance of pain helps. When the patient with Q waves also has ST segment elevation, and the onset of chest pain was abrupt and less than 6 hours earlier, he or she should be treated. At the other end of the spectrum, if pain started 20 hours earlier and is now gone, but there is some residual ST segment elevation with Q waves, we would not treat. Between these extremes it may be tough to decide so a consultation may be necessary.

ST segment depression or T wave inversion and chest pain

These changes are "nonspecific"; the patient may not have heart disease, may have angina, or could be having "non-Q wave" or subendocardial MI (Table 2.3). A few of these possibilities are surveyed in Figures 2.17–2.20.

Patients without ST segment elevation but with other ST–T wave changes who are having acute MI (the "non-Q wave" MI) fall into one of three categories: (1) the patient may actually have lateral, transmural MI with occlusion of the circumflex artery. The lateral wall often is an electrocardiographically "silent" region of the left ventricle. In theory, leads I, aVL, V5, and V6 should have typical ischemic changes. More frequently, ST seg-

Table 2.3 Causes of ST–T changes

Myocardial ischemia
LV hypertrophy
Digitalis effect
Intraventricular conduction abnormalities
(including BBB)
Early repolarization
Anoxia
Cor pulmonale
Pulmonary embolus
Myocarditis
Pericarditis
Myxedema
Hypocalemia
Hyperventilation
Nonspecific (idiopathic)
And others

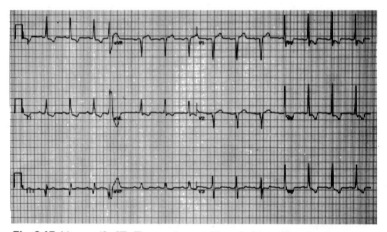

Fig. 2.17 Nonspecific ST–T wave changes. There is ST segment depression and T wave inversion in inferior and lateral leads. But this patient had no history of coronary disease or chest pain. He did have poor control of hypertension, and these ST–T wave changes may indicate early left ventricular hypertrophy.

ment elevation is not seen. Figure 2.11 is an example of acute, lateral MI with ST segment elevation, but this ECG pattern is seen in a minority of patients with lateral, transmural MI. Others without ST segment elevation may be having transmural ischemia

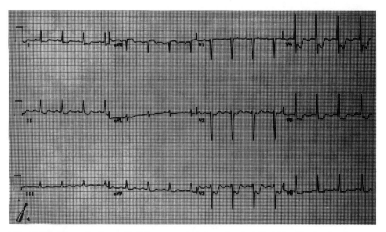

Fig. 2.18 There is dramatic ST segment depression in V3–V5 with depression also noted in inferior and lateral leads. The changes are consistent with ischemia but are not diagnostic. One problem is that the changes are "global," involving anterior plus inferior, plus lateral leads, and indicating possible acute ischemia in all three regions. But acute MI usually affects just one region. This patient was not having chest pain but was severely anoxic with impending respiratory failure. With ventilation the ST segment changes improved. Lipman and Massey have suggested that it is best to use the patient to help diagnose the ECG rather than using the ECG to diagnose the patient. You need to review the entire clinical picture.

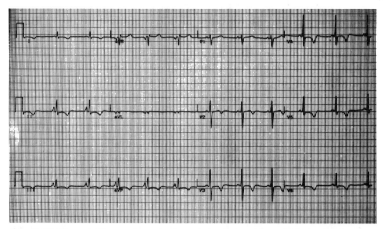

Fig. 2.19 There is T wave inversion seen in both anterior and inferior leads. Again, global rather than regional changes make us hesitate before diagnosing acute MI. This patient had no acute symptoms or history of heart disease. An ECG 3 years earlier was identical.

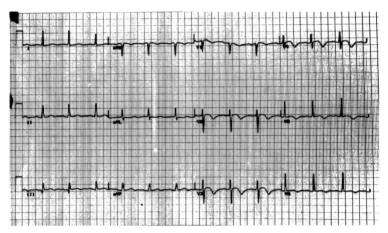

Fig. 2.20 This patient has deep, symmetrically inverted T waves across the precordial leads. This is the classical pattern for anterior, non-Q wave MI (formerly called subendocardial MI). This patient had 2 hours of chest pain but was pain-free at the time of this ECG in the emergency department. She was treated with heparin and intravenous nitroglycerin and remained stable. Angiography later in the day confirmed tight stenosis of the anterior descending artery.

and may subsequently have akinesis of the lateral wall, with CK rising above 1000 iu (our top normal is 180 iu).

(2) The ST segment depression or T wave inversion infarction may be a small MI with occlusion of a small diagonal branch of the anterior descending artery or small marginal branch of the circumflex. For such small infarctions, the patient's short-term prognosis is good without thrombolytic therapy. Long-term prognosis would be related to the extent of disease in other coronary arteries.

(3) The third type of "non-Q wave MI" should be considered a "partial" infarction. In such patients, early angiography shows a patent although tightly stenosed major coronary branch. In contrast, ST-segment-elevation MI usually means total occlusion of the artery. This non-Q wave MI causes minimal CK elevation. LV function remains good, as the bulk of ventricular myocardium served by the stenosed artery is viable. But these patients are at high risk for subsequent occlusion of the stenosed artery and their non-Q wave infarct should be considered a warning. Patients with ischemic chest pain and new, deep, and symmetrical T wave inversion in anterior precordial leads invariably are found to

have tight stenosis of the anterior descending artery (Fig. 2.20). While their symptoms respond well to heparin, aspirin, nitrates, and calcium channel blockers, they are at high risk for subsequent occlusion. Any patient with new T wave inversion in anterior leads (V1–V5) should be considered unstable and should have urgent angiography.

Whether or not to treat patients with ST segment depression, T wave inversion, and chest pain with thrombolytic agent is often uncertain. In general, we do not. Random trials have found that patients with non-ST segment elevation ("non-Q") MI have no improvement in survival with thrombolytic therapy. On the other hand, suspicion of a major MI may warrant thrombolytic therapy with nondiagnostic ST and T wave changes. This may be important for a patient with a history of prior MI or CHF. Telephone consultation with a cardiologist might be helpful for such patients.

The biggest problem with using ST segment depression and T wave changes as indicators for acute ischemia and thrombolysis is that there are so many other conditions that can cause them (Table 2.3). They are truly "nonspecific." The changes may be chronic, and it is helpful to review previous ECGs. But even new ST–T wave changes do not positively indicate ischemia. ST and T wave changes can be dynamic, varying with changes in electrolytes or drug therapy, with sleep, with fever, or with other acute illnesses.

Nonspecific ST–T wave changes are so common that patients with noncardiac pain may also have ST–T wave changes by coincidence. For example, two common illnesses, esophagitis and hypertension, may occur in the same patient causing chest discomfort and ST–T changes (Fig. 2.17). If you routinely use ST–T wave changes as an indication for thrombolytic therapy, you will treat a fair number of patients who are not having acute MI. How bad is this? Such patients are exposed to all the bleeding risks of thrombolytic therapy including intracerebral bleeding, a 0.5–1% risk. Theoretically, some will have noncardiac pain with conditions that increase the risk of dangerous bleeds such as peptic esophagitis or ulcer disease, dissection of an aortic aneurysm, pericarditis, etc. But the ISIS-2 trial found that patients with non-ST segment elevation and pain did not fare badly with thrombolytic therapy. They had no improvement in survival but at least they had no excessive risk. This trial did not compare thrombolytic therapy with aggressive treatment using heparin, aspirin, nitroglycerin, and calcium channel blockers. Our clinical experience and that of others indicates that patients with ischemia and ST segment depression respond to these measures, and this is a safer approach than thrombolytic therapy.

There is one other important thing to remember in patients with minimal ST–T wave changes. We commonly see patients who present to the emergency department with minimal ECG changes and pain that is waxing and waning. When the ECG is repeated 15 minutes later with or without a change in symptoms, dramatic ST segment elevation may have developed (Fig. 2.2). We have learned that you must repeat the ECG.

This is a simple but important clinical rule. When in doubt, repeat the ECG twice at 15–30 minute intervals. You will be surprised how often you will find that a change has occurred.

This concludes our general discussion of ECG indications for thrombolytic therapy. It is not a thorough review of ECG interpretation. Extra practice with ECG reading is provided in Appendix 2. This will include not only examples of ST segment elevation MI, but also a survey of conditions that can be misleading.

Selected reading

Aldrich HR, Wagner NB, Boswick J, *et al.* Use of initial ST-segment deviation for prediction of final electrocardiographic size of acute myocardial infarcts. Am J Cardiol 1988;61:749–53.

Goldberger AL. Myocardial Infarction. St Louis: Mosby Year Book, 1991:1–386.

GISSI. Effectiveness of thrombolytic treatment in acute myocardial infarction. Lancet 1986;1:397–402.

ISIS-2 Collaborative Group. Randomized trial of intravenous streptokinase, oral aspirin, both, or neither among 17 187 cases of suspected acute myocardial infarction: ISIS-2*. J Am Coll Cardiol 1988;12: 3–13A.

Killip T, Kimball JT. Treatment of myocardial infarction in a coronary care unit. A two year experience with 250 patients. Am J Cardiol 1967;20:457–64.

Chapter 3
Indications for treatment

Patient selection

It is a straightforward business: we weigh benefits against risks, then play the odds. That is the basis for almost every patient-management decision we make. When deciding to use thrombolytic therapy for acute MI, we are helped by large clinical trials which compare therapy with placebo (Tables 1.1, 1.2). These trials were large enough to categorize subsets of patients according to risk of MI. Not surprisingly, highest-risk patients tended to benefit most from thrombolytic therapy, and it was not possible to demonstrate benefit for low-risk patients.

For these reasons, the first step in making a decision to treat with thrombolytic agents is to evaluate the risk of the MI. Table 3.1 presents a hierachy of risk for patients with acute MI. Patients with ST segment elevation infarction and patients with acute MI with BBB have the highest mortality risk. Randomized trials have shown a definite survival benefit for thrombolytic therapy for such patients. In contrast, those with small inferior MI, ST segment depression, or T wave inversion, or those with suspected MI and no ECG changes have a lower mortality risk. The randomized trials have shown variable survival benefits with thrombolytic therapy for these patients. We consider thrombolytic therapy for the lower-risk patients only if there are mitigating clinical circumstances that increase the risk of infarction.

There are a number of such circumstances (Table 3.2). As noted in Chapter 2, Killip and Kimball found that patients with evidence for CHF or with cardiogenic shock had the highest mortality risk with acute infarction (Table 2.2). In similar fashion, clinical findings that may be associated with depressed LV function before acute MI also suggest increased risk with the fresh infarction. These would include clinical signs of heart failure, a history of MI, a history of heart failure, and possibly of long-standing hypertension. Any of these features in a setting

Table 3.1 Hierarchy of MI risk

(Highest risk; definitely treat with thrombolytic therapy)	(Lower risk; consider thrombolytic therapy based on associated conditions)
Anterior MI with ST segment elevation	Inferior MI with ST segment elevation but no reciprocal ST segment depression
Inferior MI with ST segment elevation and "reciprocal" ST segment depression	Acute MI with ST segment depression or T wave inversion
Acute MI with BBB	Suspected MI (chest pain), no ECG changes

Table 3.2 Clinical features that increase the risk of MI and would favor thrombolytic therapy

Cardiogenic shock (Killip class IV)
Pulmonary edema (Killip class III)
Rales (Killip class II)
History of prior MI
History of heart failure
History of hypertensive heart disease
RV infarct

of acute infarction would favor use of thrombolytic therapy (Table 3.2). For example, a patient with ST segment depression and typical chest pain (probable MI) who has pulmonary edema (Killip class III), should be considered for thrombolytic therapy, even without the usual ECG entry criterion (ST segment elevation).

On the other hand, there are some patients with chest pain who are at an especially high risk with thrombolytic therapy (Table 3.3). Some of these contraindications are absolute; you know that if you treat someone with intracranial bleeding who has associated T wave changes on the ECG with STK you are going to make them worse. But some of the contraindications are "relative" (Table 3.3). If a patient with a relative contraindication is having an apparently high-risk MI we would consider treating them. But if the MI appears to be low risk, a relative contraindication would influence us to avoid thrombolytic therapy.

The decision to treat thus involves balancing the clinical fea-

Table 3.3 Contraindications to thrombolytic therapy

SYNDROMES MIMICKING MI THAT CARRY
A HIGH RISK OF BLEEDING
Peptic esophagitis

Pericarditis

Aortic dissection

Intracranial bleeding with T wave changes

ABSOLUTE CONTRAINDICATIONS*
Active internal bleeding

History of cerebrovascular accident

Recent (within 2 months) intracranial or intraspinal surgery or trauma

Intracranial neoplasm, arteriovenous malformation, or aneurysm

Known bleeding diathesis

Severe uncontrolled hypertension

RELATIVE CONTRAINDICATIONS*
Recent (within 10 days) major surgery, e.g., coronary artery bypass graft, obstetrical delivery, organ biopsy, previous puncture of noncompressible vessels

Cerebrovascular disease

Recent GI or GU bleeding (within 10 days)

Recent trauma (within 10 days)

Hypertension: systolic blood pressure ≥180 mmHg and/or diastolic blood pressure ≥110 mmHg

High likelihood of left heart thrombus, e.g., mitral stenosis with atrial fibrillation

Acute pericarditis

Subacute bacterial endocarditis

Hemostatic defects including those secondary to severe hepatic or renal disease

Significant liver dysfunction

Pregnancy

Diabetic hemorrhagic retinopathy, or other hemorrhagic ophthalmic conditions

Septic thrombophlebitis or occluded AV cannula at seriously infected site

Advanced age, i.e., over 75 years old

Patients currently receiving oral anticoagulants, e.g., warfarin sodium

Any other condition in which bleeding constitutes a significant hazard or would be particularly difficult to manage because of its location

* These have been reproduced from the package inserts for rt-PA (Genentech), STK (Astra), and APSAC (Beecham).

tures in Tables 3.1, 3.2, and 3.3 when evaluating each patient. The remainder of this chapter will discuss these clinical indications and contraindications in some detail and hopefully will address the most common patient-selection issues.

Patients who definitely should be treated

As indicated in Table 3.1, patients with ST segment elevation and chest pain should be treated with thrombolytic therapy. The large placebo-controlled trials indicate a definite survival benefit for such patients who can be treated within 6 hours of the onset of pain. Patients with chest pain consistent with acute MI and BBB also had a survival benefit in these large clinical trials. It is that simple. These account for most of the patients with MI whom you will see in the emergency department. All you must be able to do is recognize ischemic chest pain and identify ST segment elevation or BBB on the ECG.

Anterior MI

Acute anterior infarction is such a bad illness that it merits additional comment. As noted, early mortality is generally caused by LV failure. Patients with first MI who have LV failure almost always have anterior MI. Patients with anterior infarction have a much lower LVEF at the time of hospital discharge, and long-term mortality is higher (Table 3.4). Although no study has specifically addressed the issue, at the Prairie Cardiovascular Center we feel that development of irreversible injury occurs more rapidly with anterior than inferior infarction. At cardiac catheterization it is our impression that patients with anterior MI who receive thrombolytic therapy 4–6 hours after onset of pain have much worse regional contractility when compared with

---

Table 3.4 Influence of MI location on survival and LVEF in survivors of Q wave MI (From Taylor, et al., 1980)

Location	30 month mortality %	% with LVEF <40%*
Anterior	28	62
Inferior	10	11

* Cardiac catheterization 12 days after MI.

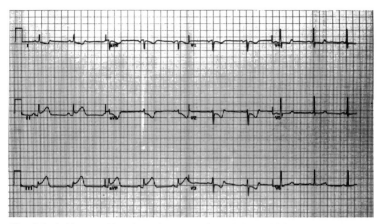

Fig. 3.1 A 46-year-old patient with acute inferior MI; this ECG was obtained 1½ hours after onset of pain. He has ST segment elevation in leads II, III, and aVF. In addition, there is marked depression of ST segments in the anterior (V1 – V4) and lateral leads (1, aVL). This reciprocal ST segment depression in anterior and lateral leads identifies this inferior MI as a large one.

patients having inferior MI. It is possible that the collateral circulation to the inferior wall is better. The anterior MI patient has less time, and you must move quickly.

Inferior MI: reciprocal ST segment depression

We do not believe that all inferior MIs are equal. The largest of the inferior MIs are those with reciprocal ST segment changes, ST segment depression in anterior or lateral leads as well as inferior ST segment elevation (Fig. 3.1). As a group, patients with reciprocal ST segment changes have occluded larger arteries supplying more muscle, have higher peak CK elevation, and have lower LVEF at the end of hospitalization (Table 3.5). We consider these higher-risk patients, and use reciprocal ST segment depression as another indicator that thrombolytic therapy is needed in an individual patient with inferior MI.

Inferior MI and hypotension

Acute inferior infarction often is accompanied by excessive vagal tone with nausea, bradycardia, and hypotension. This responds promptly to intravenous fluid replacement (normal saline is our

Table 3.5 "Reciprocal" ST segment depression in anterior leads in patients with acute inferior MI (From Gibson, et al., 1982)

	No reciprocal ST segment depression	Reciprocal ST segment depression
	(n = 21)	(n = 27)
Peak CK	653 iu	1133 iu
Predischarge LVEF	54%	46%

All differences were statistically significant.

Table 3.6 RV infarct syndrome

Setting	Acute inferior MI
Pathophysiology	Selective RV failure leads to increased right atrial pressure (RV filling pressure), low cardiac output, hypotension
Physical findings	Hypotension, jugular venous distension, pulses paradoxus (inspiratory fall >10 mmHg in systolic arterial blood pressure), little or no pulmonary congestion
Treatment	Volume expansion
Prognosis	With shock 60% survival, without hypotension >90% survival

first choice), and atropine if heart rate is low. The vagal reaction to inferior MI does not contraindicate thrombolytic therapy.

Hypotension may also indicate RV failure; the "RV infarct syndrome" (Table 3.6). This is a difficult management problem, carries a worse prognosis and, if suspected, is an indication for prompt thrombolytic therapy. These patients have selective failure of the right ventricle and hypotension, often jugular venous distension, but little pulmonary congestion. The right ventricle is not strong enough to push volume into the lungs and thus provide adequate LV filling. With inadequate filling, LV stroke volume and cardiac output fall.

The RV infarct patient has inferior ST segment elevation, and may also have increased ST segment elevation in V4R (a right chest lead, the mirror of lead V4 (Fig. 3.2). Confirmation of the diagnosis requires right heart catheterization showing high right atrial and RV diastolic pressure without elevation of pulmonary wedge pressure.

The diagnosis of RV infarct syndrome cannot be made with

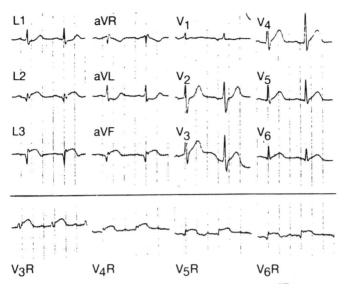

Fig. 3.2 RV infarct syndrome. Right sided precordial leads have ST segment elevation. (Reproduced with the permission of Clinical Cardiology Publishing Co, Inc, and/or the Foundation for Advances in Medicine and Science.)

certainty in the emergency department. Thrombolytic therapy should not be delayed until a pulmonary artery catheter can be inserted and hemodynamic confirmation obtained. If you suspect RV dysfunction in a patient with inferior MI, use thrombolytic therapy. Management of hypotension and the RV infarct syndrome is reviewed in Chapter 6.

In general, hypotension does not contraindicate thrombolytic therapy. All of the thrombolytic agents can produce vasodilatation and worsening of hypotension. Our general approach to the patient with hypotension has been to push fluids (normal saline) as long as the patient has no pulmonary rales, and to proceed quickly with thrombolytic therapy.

Non-ST segment elevation infarction

We have discussed ST segment depression or T wave inversion MI in Chapter 2 (also known as subendocardial, nontransmural, and/or non-Q wave infarction). Early angiography usually shows some antegrade flow in the infarct artery in contrast to patients with ST segment elevation who have total occlusion of the infarct

Table 3.7 Treatment of non-ST segment elevation MI and unstable angina pectoris

Aspirin	2 baby aspirin, chewed, then 1 adult aspirin daily (162.5–325 mg)
Heparin	5000 U i.v. bolus, then 1000–1200 U i.v. per h continuous infusion; adjust rate to maintain aPTT to 60–100 s
Intravenous nitroglycerin	Dose depends upon initial blood pressure; usually start with 10 µg/min and increase to 60–100 µg/min or to the maximum tolerated dose; watch for a fall in systolic blood pressure <100 mmHg or headache
Beta adrenergic blockers	Metoprolol 50–100 mg p.o. b.i.d. Atenolol 50–100 mg p.o. q.d. Caution: CHF, bradycardia, bronchospasm
Calcium antagonists	Diltiazem 90 mg p.o. q.i.d. effectively lowers the risk of recurrent infarction in patients with non-Q MI; it may further lower heart rate
	Nifedipine 10–20 mg p.o. q.i.d. has been especially effective in patients with angina pectoris at rest, and it has less heart rate lowering effect
	Verapamil has negative inotropic and chronotropic actions

Comment: we would use aspirin, heparin, and intravenous nitroglycerin for all patients, and add beta adrenergic blockers and calcium antagonist depending upon blood pressure and heart rate. If chest pain is not relieved in 30 minutes, consider a noncardiac diagnosis or consider thrombolytic therapy.

artery. Chest pain often responds to nitrates, aspirin, and intravenous heparin (Table 3.7). Our approach to the patient with ischemic chest pain, ST segment depression, or T wave changes is prompt use of nitroglycerin (sublingual, then intravenous), aspirin, and intravenous heparin. If that does not work and the patient continues to have pain after 30 minutes, then we consider thrombolytic therapy. If there is evidence for heart failure (Table 3.2) we would be influenced to treat with thrombolytic therapy earlier.

The ISIS-2 and GISSI-1 trials included non-ST segment elevation patients. There was no improvement in survival in the non-ST elevation patients or patients without BBB who were treated with STK (Table 3.8). But at least the risk of bleeding was no higher

Table 3.8 ECG changes and mortality with STK therapy

	Mortality (%)			
	GISSI-1		ISIS-2	
ECG changes	STK	Placebo	STK†	Placebo
ST segment elevation	10*	13	9*	13
BBB	—	—	20*	25
ST segment depression	21	16	19	19
Other	8	9	4	6
Normal ECG	—	—	2	4

* Significant improvement, $p < 0.05$.
† STK alone, not STK + aspirin.

than in other patients. Remember that these trials were comparing STK with placebo. For the non-ST segment elevation patient the trials were not comparing thrombolytic therapy with an aggressive regimen of aspirin, heparin, and intravenous nitrates (Table 3.7). Our experience is that this treatment approach works for most patients.

Typical ischemic chest pain and a normal ECG

If a patient has typical chest pain but no ECG changes, have you excluded MI? Unfortunately not. Always repeat the ECG if the history suggests MI. But even if the ECG remains normal, MI has not been excluded. It is possible to occlude some coronary branches without affecting the 12-lead ECG. Most commonly, a blocked circumflex artery supplying the lateral wall of the heart can produce either no ECG change or only minor ST–T abnormalities. Such patients may have transmural MI, some with CK rising above 1000 iu (our laboratory normal is 0–180 iu). Cardiac catheterization later shows occlusion of the circumflex artery or one of its branches and an area of akinesis in the lateral wall.

The arguments for and against treatment of patients with pain but no ECG changes parallel those outlined for patients with ST segment depression and chest pain. If you are convinced that the patient is having ischemic pain, you just need to understand that you may be wrong and could be treating noncardiac illness with a thrombolytic drug (Table 2.1). If the patient is having typical

Table 3.9 Time from onset of chest pain to STK therapy and mortality (the GISSI-1 trial, $n = 11\,806$)

Time to treatment (hrs)	Mortality (%)		
	STK	Placebo	Reduction
<1	8.2	15.4	47*
≤3[†]	9.2	12.0	23*
3–6	11.7	14.1	17*
6–9	12.6	14.1	11
9–12	15.8	13.6	—

* A significant reduction in mortality, $p < 0.05$.
† Separate survival statistics for patients treated at 2–3 hours not available.

ischemic pain and has evidence for heart failure, we might be influenced in favor of treatment with thrombolytic therapy.

Unstable angina pectoris

Unstable angina is a pattern of waxing and waning chest pain which can be mistaken for MI. ST segment changes may be transient and are often reversed by nitroglycerin. With unstable angina, ST segment elevation is less common than ST segment depression and T wave inversion. Thrombolytic therapy has been advocated by some, and it does work to stabilize these acutely ill patients with chest pain. But patients with unstable angina also have symptom relief with heparin, nitrates, beta blockers, and calcium antagonists (Table 3.7), and this approach carries a lower risk of major bleeding complications or stroke. Presently, we do not believe that unstable angina indicates a need for thrombolytic therapy.

Time to treatment

The randomized trials have all compared patients who were treated 6–24 hours after onset of MI with patients treated earlier. Maximum survival and LV function benefits come with early treatment (Table 3.9). We will discuss early treatment at length in Chapter 10, where it is shown that the most important thing that you can do to help your patients is to shorten time to therapy.

Unlike the GISSI-1 trial, ISIS-2 found that thrombolytic therapy for patients treated 6–12 hours from onset of pain had a small but demonstrable survival benefit. ISIS-2 also found a survival benefit for patients treated 13–24 hours after onset of MI. So what should be done? We try to individualize and estimate relative benefits and risks for the given patient. If the patient is later in the course of MI (6–24 hours), appears to be having a high-risk infarction (Table 3.2), and has no contraindications to thrombolytic therapy, we would provide treatment. If it looks like a low-risk MI, or there are relative contraindications, we would not treat with thrombolytic drugs. There will be times when you are uncertain: this is another time for consultation.

Another important issue is whether there are increased risks of thrombolytic therapy if it is given late. The risk of bleeding (GI, urinary tract, cerebral) appears to be no greater with therapy administered late in the course of MI. On the other hand, there are suggestive data indicating that the risk of myocardial rupture is higher in patients who are treated more than 12 hours after the onset of chest pain. Risk of myocardial rupture may be higher if patients have been on steroid therapy. This risk may be lowered by the adjunctive use of beta blockers (Chapter 8).

Advanced age and thrombolysis

Our early studies of thrombolytic therapy excluded patients above 75 years old. This was the case with a number of the randomized trials as well (Table 1.1). But both the ISIS-2 and the GISSI-1 trials, comparing STK with placebo, had no age limitation. Not only did these studies show a survival benefit for elderly patients, they found that the survival benefit was greater than it was for younger patients.

This should come as no surprise. Older patients have a higher morbidity and mortality risk with any illness. If you wish to demonstrate benefits for any treatment, study highest-risk patients. For example, patients with coronary artery disease and poor LV function have the worst prognosis. Because of the high risk with medical therapy, randomized studies of bypass surgery have shown that patients with poor LV function have the greatest survival benefit even though they have higher surgical mortality. Similarly, elderly patients have the highest mortality risk with MI. A survival benefit with thrombolytic therapy for these patients was clear in both GISSI-1 and ISIS-2 (Table 3.10).

This does not mean that all or even most old people do well.

Table 3.10 Elderly patients and early mortality after thrombolytic therapy

			Mortality, deaths/total (%)	
Trial	Drug	Age group	Drug	Placebo
GISSI-1	STK	≤65	217/3824 (5%)	291/3784 (7%)*
		66–75	240/1444 (16%)	261/1442 (18%)
		>75	171/592 (29%)	206/623 (33%)
ISIS-2	STK†	<60	162/3864 (4%)	224/3856 (6%)*
		60–69	320/3033 (11%)	435/3023 (14%)*
		≥70	309/1695 (18%)	370/1716 (22%)*
ASSET	rt-PA	≤55	29/748 (4%)	33/745 (4%)
		56–65	63/963 (7%)	71/896 (8%)
		66–75	90/827 (11%)	140/852 (16%)*
AIMS	APSAC	<65	21/405 (5%)	35/411 (9%)
		≥65	11/90 (12%)	26/86 (30%)*

* Significant difference, $p < 0.05$.
† STK alone, not STK + aspirin.

On the contrary, they have much higher cardiac and noncardiac morbidity after thrombolytic therapy. Problematic hematoma following arterial cannulation or venipuncture are more common in older patients. Stroke is more common in elderly patients. Elderly patients seem to have a greater "early hazard." That is to say, more of them die in the first day after MI with thrombolytic therapy. Most of these deaths are cardiac and due to LV failure (not to complications). After the first day the survival curves for elderly patients treated with STK diverge dramatically from those treated with placebo.

We now treat elderly patients with thrombolytic therapy without hesitation. But in this population we are especially careful to look for contraindications to therapy. As with any therapy in medicine, careful patient selection can be equated with good clinical judgment. We tend to avoid thrombolytic therapy for elderly patients who are frail, debilitated, or who have other medical problems.

Chest pain has resolved but ST segment elevation persists

We commonly see patients who have symptoms wax and wane early in the course of infarction. If the onset of chest pain is

Table 3.11 Influence of prior MI on survival and LVEF in 102 survivors of MI (From Taylor, *et al.*, 1980)

	30 month mortality (%)	Percentage LVEF <40%*
Prior MI	41	43
No prior MI	6	22

* Cardiac catheterization 12 days after MI.

within 6 hours, ST segment elevation persists, and you are convinced the chest discomfort is ischemic, use thrombolytic therapy. Chest pain will often worsen, and you will be glad you treated the patient. On the other hand, if there was chest pain all night, and it has resolved the next morning, we would be less likely to use thrombolytic therapy even with persistent ST segment elevation. This sounds more like a completed MI. As noted above, patients treated late in the course of infarction with thrombolytic agents may have higher risk of myocardial rupture.

Patients with previous MI

All studies of the natural history of MI find that patients with multiple MI have the highest mortality risk (Table 3.11). Myocardial injury is cumulative, and patients with multiple infarctions are more likely to have depressed LV function because functional reserve has been used up. For these reasons we believe patients with acute MI who have a history of prior infarction should be treated with thrombolytic therapy. A remote history of MI (with mature LV scar) does not increase the risk of thrombolytic therapy in a setting of fresh infarction.

Persistent chest pain and Q waves on the ECG

In the absence of thrombolytic therapy Q waves take hours to appear. With early reperfusion Q waves may develop over a period of minutes (Fig. 3.3). Occasionally, patients with persistent ST segment elevation and active pain will also have Q waves. It is possible that such patients had occlusion, reperfusion, then reocclusion. Q waves may thus develop early with ST segment elevation and pain that comes and goes depending upon the state of the infarct artery. It is a dynamic process. We do not consider

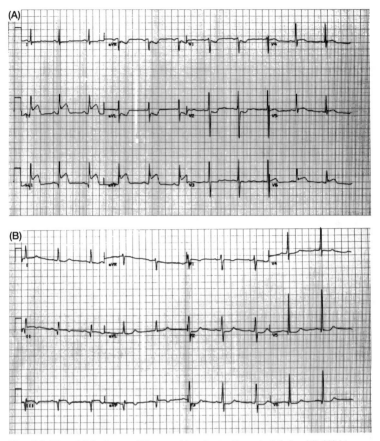

Fig. 3.3 Two ECGs from a 57-year-old patient with acute inferior MI. (A) He had improvement in chest pain and the second ECG (B) was obtained 1½ hours later. Note the development of Q waves in the inferior leads during this short interval.

Q waves a contraindication to thrombolytic therapy. On the other hand, another possibility is that Q waves may indicate that the patient is further into the course of infarction than you initially thought. Symptoms and the ECG must be considered together.

Early repolarization

Many healthy people have ST segment elevation in multiple leads, the pattern of "early repolarization." This is a frequent source of confusion in the emergency room. It commonly is seen in young patients, and especially thin young athletes with few risk factors for coronary artery disease. But early repolarization may also be seen in older patients in the "coronary age group." The magnitude of ST segment elevation is usually less than 0.2 mV (2 mm). As with pericarditis, changes may be diffuse and involve more than one myocardial region (i.e. ST segment changes in inferior and anterior leads). And like pericarditis, the ST segments retain their upward concavity (Fig. 2.12). Because early repolarization is a common finding, it may occur coincidentally in patients with noncardiac chest pain syndromes.

Contraindications to thrombolytic therapy

Contraindications cannot be considered alone, but must be weighed with the patient's clinical presentation. There are some contraindications that are so absolute you would never consider thrombolytic therapy. These would include active bleeding, or recent stroke (Table 3.3). With some other contraindications, you might "bend" if the patient appeared to be having an especially high-risk MI. In the face of a small, low-risk infarction, even a relative contraindication may be enough to influence you not to treat with thrombolytic therapy. Table 3.3 outlines the contraindications to thrombolytic therapy: this is the FDA approved list of contraindications. In addition to these contraindications which indicate a higher risk for bleeding complications, we have added conditions which cause chest pain that may be difficult to distinguish from MI (Table 2.1) and would be disastrous if treated with thrombolytic drugs.

Conditions causing chest pain that contraindicate thrombolytic therapy

Pericarditis
The major risk in treating pericarditis with thrombolytic agents is bleeding into the pericardium and cardiac tamponade. Acute pericarditis often occurs in young people who have few risk factors for premature coronary disease (Table 3.12). It may be accompanied by symptoms such as fever or cough that indicate viral illness. The pain with pericarditis often is sharp, not typically "ischemic" in quality. It may be pleuritic and may be positional. An occasional patient will mention pain with swallowing. Physical

Table 3.12 Clinical features of chest pain syndromes

	Acute MI	Pericarditis	Aortic dissection
Frequency	Common	Less common	Less common
Pain	Midchest, typically "ischemic," dull, heavy	Midchest, pleuritic may vary with position or swallowing, sharp	Midchest, "tearing," radiation to back
Associated conditions	Risk factors for ischemic heart disease	Cough, fever, "viral illness"	History of hypertension, loss of pulses, neurological changes
ECG	Regional ST segment elevation, upwardly convex or flat ST segments	Diffuse, global ST segment elevation, upwardly concave ST segments	Nonspecific ST segment changes or LV hypertrophy pattern
Other findings	Increased cardiac enzymes	Increased sedimentation rate, pericardial effusion on echo (variable), friction rub	Wide mediastinum on chest X-ray, dissection on echo (variable), difference in blood pressure in arms

examination often reveals a pericardial friction rub; in the presence of a friction rub we would be reluctant to use thrombolytic agents. There may be ST segment elevation on the ECG, but the changes may be different than those seen with infarction (Fig. 3.4). With pericarditis, ST segment elevation is more diffuse, involving ECG leads reflecting multiple vascular distributions. ST segment elevation with acute ischemia tends to be regional, involving just one vascular distribution. It would be unusual for a patient to occlude arteries to both anterior and inferior walls simultaneously. The ST segments, although elevated, retain the normal upward concavity with pericarditis (Fig. 2.12).

At times it is hard to be sure. There are no laboratory tests that are specific for pericarditis. The sedimentation rate is often elevated. The echocardiogram may or may not demonstrate pericardial effusion. But both the echocardiogram and sedimentation rate are worth checking in the borderline case, even if you finally decide the patient is having MI and elect to go ahead with thrombolytic therapy. Abnormal results might influence subsequent therapy.

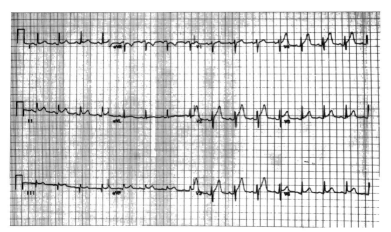

Fig. 3.4 A 32-year-old patient with chest pain lasting most of the day. He also had mild fever and cough. Pain was pleuritic in quality. This ECG shows ST segment elevation in anterior leads (V2–V6) as well as inferior leads (II, III, and aVF). It would be highly unlikely for him to have simultaneous infarction of both anterior and inferior walls (which would require simultaneous occlusion of two different arteries). In addition ST segments are upwardly concave. The correct diagnosis is acute pericarditis (based upon clinical findings plus ECG changes).

Suspected dissecting aortic aneurysm

This most commonly occurs in older patients with a history of hypertension. The pain often has a "tearing" quality and it may radiate through to the back (Table 3.12). Physical examination may show a difference in blood pressure in the arms. Neurologic symptoms may develop if the dissection involves major branches from the aortic arch. Of course, neurologic symptoms or signs would be strong contraindications to thrombolytic therapy.

It is possible for the intimal flap to occlude a coronary ostium during aortic dissection. This would cause true MI with typical chest pain and ST segment elevation. In our series of 1012 patients we encountered one such patient who had inferior MI, but at catheterization (after thrombolytic therapy) was found to have dissection of the ascending aorta, occlusion of the right coronary ostium, and a normal distal right coronary artery. Although this combination of events can lead to the inadvertent use of thrombolytic therapy, it will be unusually rare.

We generally discourage getting a chest X-ray before ordering thrombolytic therapy as it unnecessarily delays treatment. But if you are concerned about aortic dissection, a chest X-ray before treatment makes sense. Look for widening of the mediastinum.

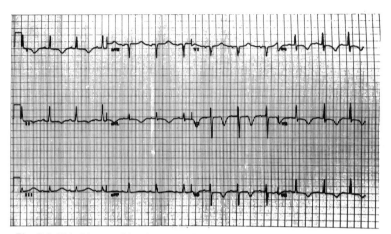

Fig. 3.5 This 64-year-old patient was obtunded and had no history of acute chest pain. The ECG shows symmetrical and deep T wave inversion in leads V2–V6, I, II, aVL. The QT interval is prolonged. A CT (computed tomography) scan subsequently documented subarachnoid hemorrhage. Such ECG changes are commonly seen in patients with intracranial bleeding. It is important to treat the patient, not the ECG; neurological symptoms are a strong contraindication to thrombolytic therapy.

If you routinely treat patients with chest pain and ST segment depression and T wave inversion, you will be more likely to inadvertently treat patients with aortic dissection. In the ASSET trial, five such patients were treated who were subsequently found to have aortic dissection, and all five died. The mortality risk of ascending aortic dissection is unusually high anyway, but as a rule we prefer to avoid holding the "smoking gun." It is one more reason we reserve thrombolytic therapy for patients with ST segment elevation or BBB infarction; we are less likely to inadvertently treat patients with noncardiac etiologies of chest pain such as aortic dissection.

When clinical history is uncertain, and you are concerned about pericarditis or dissection but cannot exclude MI, another approach is urgent angiography. If the patient is having MI, direct angioplasty is possible (Chapter 7).

Intracranial bleeding and injury
Patients with intracranial bleeding including subarachnoid hemorrhage may develop deep T wave inversion on the ECG (Fig. 3.5). The T wave changes on the ECG do not come from the head,

they come from the heart. Myocardial CK (CK-MB) may be slightly elevated, and autopsy studies have shown subendocardial myelysis. Apparently brain injury can provoke myocardial injury, probably via sympathetic discharge and vascular spasm. This may occur with normal coronary arteries; there is low risk for further myocardial injury. ST segment elevation is rate. These patients tend not to have chest discomfort, and neurological symptoms are usually present. Thrombolytic therapy is seldom an issue.

Other contraindications

The current FDA approved guidelines are reproduced in Table 3.3. "Active bleeding" is an "absolute" contraindication, but "bleeding within 10 days" is considered a "relative" contraindication. We have perhaps been more conservative in our clinical practice and offer these observations:

GI or urinary tract bleeding

Recent ($\leq$2 weeks) or active bleeding in the GI or GU tract is a red flag. Our experience is that patients with recent bleeding almost certainly will bleed when given thrombolytic therapy. The only difference is that the bleeding will be worse than it was originally. With a clinical history of more remote bleeding, the risk with thrombolytic therapy falls. A patient with peptic ulcer disease years earlier, without bleeding and with no recent symptoms would be a fair candidate for thrombolytic therapy. A remote (more than 2 years previous) history of bleeding from ulcer disease and no recent symptoms would not contraindicate thrombolysis but does identify a minimally higher risk. Bleeding 1–2 months previously, is a grey zone, and the decision to treat may depend on the risk of the MI (Tables 3.1, 3.2). Any patient with a history of dyspepsia or ulcer disease should have aggressive antacid treatment.

The potential for recurrent bleeding may be apparent from the history. For example, a patient with a history of GU bleeding who still has his kidney stone is at higher risk than one who has had surgical correction.

Invasive procedures

Recent surgery is a contraindication to thrombolytic therapy. Physicians and surgeons often are tempted to treat the hospitalized patient with postoperative infarction. The patient is right there, the diagnosis is made rapidly, and there is an element of guilt (the MI happended while under their care). If there has been surgery within 2 weeks you can count on major bleeding. If surgery occurred 3–6 weeks earlier the risk of bleeding is also high, and the decision to treat should be related to the risk of the MI. We are comfortable with thrombolytic treatment more than 6 weeks after surgery. Patients who have had invasive, albeit nonsurgical procedures including percutaneous biopsies of lung, pleura, liver, or kidney are at equally high risk for major bleeding. Would you consider thrombolytic therapy for a patient who has had cardiac catheterization? Possibly, since bleeding could be contained with local compression. The ability to control a bleeding site enters into the assessment of risk.

Patients with postoperative ST segment elevation MI may be good candidates for urgent cardiac catheterization and possible angioplasty. The success rate for primary angioplasty is quite good, and morbidity is low, even for these postoperative patients.

Stroke and TIA

The risk of intracranial hemorrhage is increased in patients with prior history of stroke or TIA and in elderly patients. This complication is often fatal and always catastrophic. Associated conditions which increase the risk of intracranial hemorrhage including severe, uncontrolled hypertension, vague neurologic symptoms, unexplained recent headache, head trauma, or history of prior stroke or TIA are good reasons to avoid thrombolytic therapy. This should be well documented in the medical record and this is another time for second opinion, consultation.

Hypertension

A history of poorly-controlled hypertension is a contraindication to thrombolytic therapy because of the increased risk for intracranial bleeding. Patients often respond to chest pain, or any pain, with an increase in blood pressure. However, if repeat blood pressure measurements show persistent elevation of systolic pressure above 200 mmHg or diastolic blood pressure above 110 mmHg, avoid thrombolytic treatment. Patients with borderline elevation of blood pressure, who have the pressure fall into the acceptable range with intravenous beta blocker or nitroglycerin therapy can be treated with thrombolytic agents.

Coagulation disorders

Patients with coagulation disorders including thrombocytopenia are at higher risk for bleeding, but the risk appears related to the severity of the disorder. A patient with a factor deficiency who also has a history of bleeding is at a higher risk than one who has mild factor deficiency without prior bleeding. A borderline low platelet count is not a contraindication to treatment.

As thrombolytic therapy was being developed, and we were all slightly timid, a number of centers did coagulation studies before starting therapy. This is not necessary. In the absence of a bleeding diathesis history, it is unnecessary to wait for the prothrombin time, partial thromboplastin time, or platelet count before starting thrombolytic therapy. In fact, we consider it an error as it substantially delays treatment (Chapter 10).

Cardiopulmonary resuscitation (CPR)

In our experience, patients with acute infarction who have VF and brief periods of CPR may be treated with thrombolytic agents with reasonable safety. On the other hand, when CPR is prolonged or when there is obvious chest wall trauma during CPR, there is a higher risk for bleeding. If the MI is a high risk one (Tables 3.1, 3.2), we would consider thrombolytic therapy.

Diabetic retinopathy

There have been no systematic studies indicating a higher risk of bleeding in patients with diabetic retinopathy. Our ophthalmology colleagues indicate it is a definite possibility. Because of the rarity of the condition, we expect that anecdotal information will accumulate, and we will have more definite guidelines in the future. At present, we agree with the designation of retinopathy as a relative contraindication, and would recommend thrombolytic therapy only for those patients with high-risk MI. This would be a situation where outside consultation (perhaps with the ophthalmologist as well as your cardiology consultant) would be helpful.

Menstruation

MI is uncommon in women during the childbearing years. We have treated a handful of women in their 30s and 40s who were menstruating. Excessive bleeding has not been a problem, but we recognize its potential. Excessive menstrual bleeding can be attenuated with hormonal therapy making it possible to treat the menstruating patient with high-risk MI. We personally would not consider thrombolytic therapy for women who are pregnant or within 1 month postpartum, but are aware of no data addressing this situation.

Anticoagulation therapy
Some clinical trials have included warfarin therapy as a contraindication to entering patients. We would treat patients on warfarin who appear to be having high-risk infarction. Aspirin therapy is not considered a contraindication.

Prior thrombolytic therapy
Previous use of thrombolytic drugs is not a contraindication to treatment. Those who have been treated with STK or APSAC or who have had streptococcal infection in the previous 6 months will have antibodies to STK. This increases the chance of an allergic reaction to STK and APSAC. Antibodies may also bind these drugs and thus reduce effectiveness. Such patients should be treated with rt-PA, a native protein and thus nonantigenic.

Advanced age
In earlier discussion we indicated that elderly patients may have a greater survival benefit with thrombolytic therapy for acute MI than younger patients. Advanced age is thus not an absolute contraindication to treatment. On the other hand, clinical judgment must be exercised. The older patients may be at higher risk for bleeding complications and particularly for intracranial hemorrhage. Look carefully for any contraindication to treatment. It does not appear sensible to treat elderly patients who are especially frail or who have other serious medical illnesses.

General observations on patient selection and contraindications

We physicians are basically conservative about new and especially dangerous therapies. The complications of thrombolytic therapy are potentially catastrophic; there is no way to minimize that fact. In addition, complications occur frequently enough that you will encounter them in your practice.

From early in our training we were taught that the first rule in medicine is to avoid harming our patients. It is still an important rule, but we also recognize that most modern therapies carry risks. That is true for antibiotic therapy for infectious diseases, heparin therapy for pulmonary embolus, and all surgical therapies. Even if you limit your practice to holistic medicine, encouraging good diet and exercise, you will provoke guilt feelings and anxiety in some patients.

Thrombolytic therapy, like all medical practice, involves risks. But we now have adequate data to weigh the risks against potential benefits. The results are clear: MI is a dangerous illness, and thrombolytic therapy reduces that danger. With this background we offer a new motto: forget *primum non nocere*, play the best odds.

Selected reading

Caplin JL. Acute right ventricular infarction. BMJ 1989;299:69–70.

Gibson RS, Crampton RS, Watson DD, *et al*. Precordial ST-segment depression during acute inferior myocardial infarction: Clinical, scintigraphic and angiographic correlations. Circulation 1982;66: 732–41.

GISSI. Effectiveness of thrombolytic treatment in acute myocardial infarction. Lancet 1986;1:397–402.

ISIS-2 Collaborative Group. Randomized trial of intravenous streptokinase, oral aspirin, both, or neither among 17 187 cases of suspected acute myocardial infarction: ISIS-2*. J Am Coll Cardiol 1988;12: 3–13A.

Isner JM. Right ventricular myocardial infarction. JAMA 1988;259: 712–18.

Killip T, Kimball JT. Treatment of myocardial infarction in a coronary care unit. A two year experience with 250 patients. Am J Cardiol 1967;20:457–64.

Taylor GJ, Humphries JO, Mellits ED, *et al*. Predictors of clinical course, coronary anatomy and left ventricular function after recovery from acute myocardial infarction. Circulation 1980;62:960–70.

Wilcox RG, Von der Lippe G, Olsson CG, Jensen G, Skene AM, Hampton JR. Trial of tissue plasminogen activator for mortality reduction in acute myocardial infarction. Anglo-Scandinavian study of early thrombolysis (ASSET). Lancet 1988;2:525–30.

Chapter 4
Pharmacology of thrombolytic agents

Fibrinolysis

Injury to the wall of blood vessels exposes collagen, activates platelets, and stimulates formation of a platelet plug. This in turn triggers the clotting cascade whose end product is thrombin, a protease that mediates conversion of fibrinogen to fibrin. Fibrin is the insoluble, noncellular, fibrous component of thrombus. This sequence of events is responsible for production of a hemostatic plug at the site of a punctured vessel, but also for formation of pathologic thrombus on the ulcerated surface of atheromatous plaque (Fig. 4.1).

Clot formation and clot lysis are in dynamic equilibrium. When thrombus forms, its size must be limited; thrombus cannot be allowed to propagate indefinitely. Thrombus forming in blood vessels must be removed to restore patency. This is the role of the thrombolytic, or fibrinolytic system. As soon as thrombus forms, the fibrinolytic system is activated.

The fibrinolytic system works at three sites (Fig. 4.1): the hemostatic plug, interluminal thrombus, and circulating fibrinogen. Fibrinogenolysis is initiated by plasminogen activators, compounds which convert the zymogen, plasminogen, to the active, fibrinolytic enzyme, plasmin. Plasmin, in turn, digests fibrin, breaking it into fibrin degradation products (Fig. 4.2). Plasminogen activators include the endogenous compounds UK and t-PA, as well as exogenous, foreign compounds such as STK and APSAC.

Plasminogen is found in the circulation in a "free" state. As clot forms, it is incorporated into the thrombus and is bound to fibrin. The ideal thrombolytic drug or plasminogen activator would move directly into the thrombus and work only on fibrin-bound plasminogen. But the thrombolytic agent activates circulating plasminogen as well, producing circulating plasmin and the so-called "lytic state" (Fig. 4.2). Free plasmin in the circulation

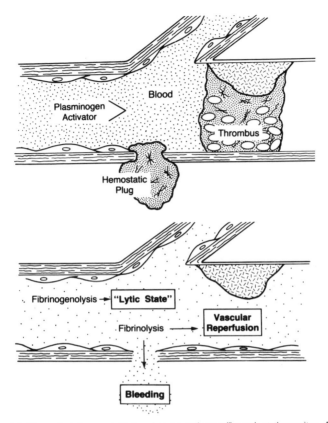

Fig. 4.1 Thrombolytic agents ("plasminogen activators") work at three sites. At all three sites the basic reaction is the conversion of plasminogen to plasmin, the enzyme which actively digests fibrinogen. This reaction takes place in thrombi including hemostatic plug and intraluminal thrombus that forms at sites of deep arterial injury. The intraluminal thrombus may be occlusive and is considered pathologic. The third site of activity is free plasminogen in the circulation which is converted to free plasmin. This in turn digests fibrinogen producing a hypocoagulable state. (From Marder VJ, Sherry S. N Engl J Med 1988;318:1516.)

digests, and therefore depletes circulating fibrinogen and other clotting factors producing a hypocoagulable state. In addition, the fibrinogen degradation products ("split products") have anticoagulant activity.

Whether a drug works primarily on circulating or fibrin-bound plasminogen, depends on a number of factors. The first is the affinity of the drug for fibrin. *In vitro* studies have shown that all

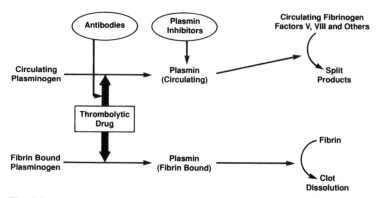

Fig. 4.2 Many things can happen to divert the thrombolytic agent while it is "on its way to work." What you want it to do is get into the clot and activate fibrin-bound plasminogen. This leads to prompt clot dissolution. But in varying degrees, the drugs also work on circulating plasminogen, producing free plasmin. This free plasmin, in turn, can also dissolve thrombus, and high levels of circulating plasmin and fibrinogen depletion constitute the "lytic state." Plasmin inhibitors may neutralize circulating plasmin. Antibodies may neutralize STK and APSAC. Basically, all of these systems must be saturated before there is adequate thrombolytic drug "left over" to reach clot-bound plasminogen.

the thrombolytic agents, except UK, readily move into thrombus (Fig. 4.3). But among the drugs there is a variation in the degree of fibrin affinity. APSAC was engineered to have fibrin affinity exceeding that of STK, and rt-PA has strong fibrin affinity.

A second determinant of the clot-specific activity of a plasminogen activator is the availability of the drug at the level of thrombus (Fig. 4.2). Circulating antibodies to both STK and APSAC bind and thus inactivate a share of these agents. In addition, circulating plasminogen is in competition with fibrin-bound plasminogen for the drug. As there is a rough equilibrium, agents which are active in the circulation must be given in a sufficient quantity to saturate circulating plasminogen and antibodies so that there is drug available at the level of thrombus. Stated differently, the "gradient for diffusion" of the drug into the thrombus is greater for agents that are less active in the circulation (and are thus not "neutralized" in the circulation).

The fibrinolytic system is modulated by inhibitors (Fig. 4.2). The most prominent inhibitor is alpha$_2$ antiplasmin, which rapidly neutralizes plasmin within the vascular space and serves to keep active plasmin levels low in the circulation. Alpha$_2$ antiplasmin binds to the same plasmin sites that bind plasmin to fibrin. Thus,

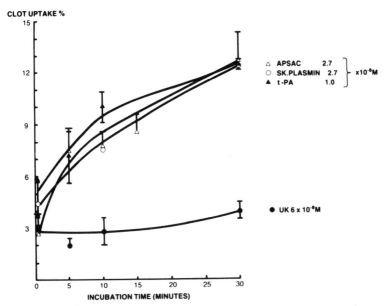

CLOT UPTAKE %

△ APSAC	2.7
○ SK.PLASMIN	2.7	× 10⁻⁸M
▲ t-PA	1.0

● UK 6 x 10⁻⁸M

INCUBATION TIME (MINUTES)

Fig. 4.3 Uptake of thrombolytic drugs into preformed clots. This *in vitro* study showed that APSAC, STK, and rt-PA are readily incorporated into preformed thrombus. UK, because of its low affinity for fibrin, is not incorporated into thrombus. (From Ferres H. Drugs 1987;33(Suppl 3):52.)

plasmin that is bound to fibrin cannot be inactivated by circulating alpha$_2$ antiplasmin. Drugs that are active in the circulation (STK, UK, APSAC), must generate enough plasmin to "saturate" alpha$_2$ antiplasmin, leaving adequate quantities of both drug and plasmin for action at the tissue level.

Lytic state

When enough circulating plasmin is produced to overwhelm inhibitors, the uninhibited free plasmin produces a systemic lytic state. Not only is this plasmin available for action at the tissue level, but the circulating plasmin also degrades fibrinogen and clotting factors V, VIII, and others (Fig. 4.2). Systemically acting thrombolytic agents reduce circulating fibrinogen levels to <15% of baseline. Systemic fibrinogenolysis and fibrinogen depletion produce a hypocoagulable state, thus reducing the risk of rethrombosis. Fibrin degradation products inhibit both platelet function and other clotting mechanism, and so have an anti-

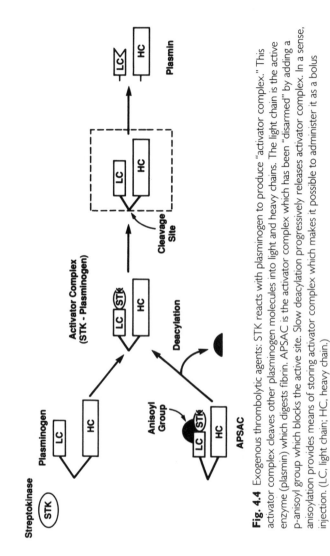

Fig. 4.4 Exogenous thrombolytic agents: STK reacts with plasminogen to produce "activator complex." This activator complex cleaves other plasminogen molecules into light and heavy chains. The light chain is the active enzyme (plasmin) which digests fibrin. APSAC is the activator complex which has been "disarmed" by adding a p-anisoyl group which blocks the active site. Slow deacylation progressively releases activator complex. In a sense, anisoylation provides means of storing activator complex which makes it possible to administer it as a bolus injection. (LC, light chain; HC, heavy chain.)

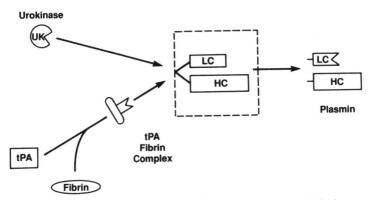

Fig. 4.5 Endogenous thrombolytic agents: UK is an active enzyme which cleaves the plasminogen molecule. It is commonly found in urine. t-PA requires fibrin as a cofactor before it is enzymatically active.

coagulant action. For these reasons, agents working systemically to deplete fibrinogen may add an element of protection in the 24–36 hours after thrombolytic therapy. This is one explanation for the lower incidence of arterial reocclusion after treatment with agents that deplete fibrinogen (i.e., that work systemically in the circulation, and not just at the "tissue" or clot level). The low fibrinogen level persists as long as the active drug is present, then progressively returns to normal over 36–48 hours.

Prothrombotic effect

Most of the thrombolytic agents also activate platelets and other clotting mechanisms, a paradoxical prothrombotic effect. If the process of thrombolysis is interrupted, rebound thrombosis may occur.

Thrombolytic agents

While each of the thrombolytic agents ultimately promotes conversion of plasminogen to plasmin, each has a different mechanism of action (Figs 4.4, 4.5). Plasminogen is composed of a light chain and a heavy chain. When the thrombolytic agent (or "plasminogen activator") removes the heavy chain by cleaving a single bond, the light chain (plasmin) assumes a configuration that is able to digest fibrin.

Table 4.1 Thrombolytic drugs: pharmacology and clinical features

	STK	APSAC	rt-PA	UK
Half-life (min)	23	90	4	16
Speed of fibrinolysis	2+	3+	4+	2+
Fibrin enhancement	2+	2+	4+	1+
90 min patency (Treatment @4.8 hrs)‡	31%	NA	62%	NA
90 min patency* (Treatment within 3 hrs)	60–65%	65–70%	65–70%	60–70%
24-h patency	80–90%	80–90%	80–90%	NA
Reocclusion	15%	10%	20%	10%
Fibrinogenolysis	4+	4+	2+	3+
Bleeding	4+	4+	4+	4+
CNS bleed§	0.5%	0.6%	0.7%	NA
Allergic side effects	Yes	Yes	No	No
Hypotension	2+	3+	1+	2+
AWP†	$186	$2011	$2640	$287

2+ slight; 3+ moderate, 4+ severe.

* From Marder and Sherry, 1988.

† Average wholesale price (AWP) to the hospital. Our hospital purchases STK at a discount price of $79, APSAC for $1649; there has been no discount for rt-PA.

‡ From TIMI-1; patients treated 4.8 hours after onset of MI (see test).

§ From ISIS-3 which used subcutaneous heparin for the majority of patients; with intravenous heparin the risk is higher.

STK and APSAC are exogenous agents, not naturally occurring. Both UK and t-PA are endogenous proteins. A summary of clinical actions of the thrombolytic agents is found in Table 4.1.

STK

STK is a protein generated by beta-hemolytic streptococci. STK itself is not an enzyme but instead forms a complex with either plasminogen or plasmin (Fig. 4.4). The STK–plasminogen or STK–plasmin complexes work to cleave other plasminogen molecules producing more plasmin. As STK has an affinity for fibrin, it works at the level of thrombus (on fibrin-bound plasminogen) as well as in the circulation. The plasmin that is produced in the circulation is inhibited by alpha$_2$ antiplasmin. As noted above, large enough doses of STK must be infused to produce enough plasmin to saturate circulating alpha$_2$ antiplasmin. Excess plasmin (that which is not inhibited), is both thrombolytic and fibrinogenolytic.

Since STK works on free, circulating plasminogen, a sufficiently high dose is also needed to "saturate" circulating plasminogen. In a sense, plasminogen in the thrombus is competing with circulating plasminogen for STK (Fig. 4.2).

Low fibrinogen levels and depletion of clotting factors V, VIII, and others, produce a hypocoagulable state after STK therapy. In addition, fibrin degradation products work as anticoagulants, inhibiting platelet aggregation, and fibrinogen polymerization. The fibrinogen level is near zero for 2–4 hours following STK infusion and then gradually returns to normal over 24–36 hours (the time it takes for the liver to generate fibrinogen and other clotting factors).

After injection of STK there is a rapid clearance phase (half-life of 18 minutes) which is followed by a slower clearance (half-life of 80 minutes). The rapid early clearance probably comes from neutralization of STK by antibodies, a result of prior streptococcal infection. Antibody levels vary from patient to patient. Although it has not been documented clinically, higher levels of antibody in patients recently treated with STK theoretically make its reuse within 6 months unwise. Instead we use rt-PA for patients with recurrent MI who have previously been treated with STK.

Another effect of STK (and other plasminogen activators) is transient hypotension shortly after infusion. This is mediated by the generation of kallikrein which converts kinogen to bradykinin. Bradykinin is a vasodilator. The resulting hypotension usually responds to volume replacement and a reduced rate of STK infusion. It is rare that the drug has to be stopped because of hypotension.

APSAC

APSAC was engineered based upon knowledge that the STK–plasminogen complex is the active agent which cleaves the light and heavy chains of plasminogen. The goal in producing this new compound was to increase duration of action, stability in the

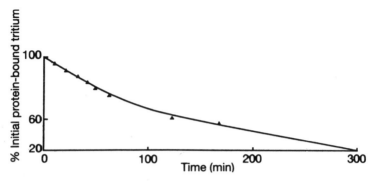

Fig. 4.6 After a bolus injection of tritium-labeled APSAC, there is progressive loss of protein-bound tritium which indicates deacylation. The half-life in whole blood is 106 minutes. (From Clinical Cardiology Publishing Co, Inc, and/or the Foundation for Advances in Medicine and Science.)

circulation, fibrin binding, and speed of thrombolysis. Each of these goals has been achieved with APSAC.

The site on APSAC which cleaves the bond between the light and heavy chains of plasminogen is temporarily disarmed by an anisoyl group tagged to the compound by a reversible acylating agent (Fig. 4.4). This inactivated complex can be injected as a bolus. Deacylation of APSAC results in "slow release" of activator complex (Fig. 4.6). Active compound is thus maintained in the circulation for a longer period than with any of the other thrombolytic agents. The half-life of APSAC, determined by the rate of deacylation, is about 90–100 minutes, but a significant quantity of APSAC may still be present after 4–5 hours.

In addition to longer activity in the circulation, APSAC is also more active than STK at the level of thrombus. There are two reasons. The first is that the fibrin-binding site on the heavy chain of APSAC has been modified to increase its affinity to fibrin. The second is improved diffusion of the drug into thrombus. After infusion of STK, there is competition between circulating plasminogen and thrombus for the drug. With APSAC, there is no plasminogen binding of the anisoylated compound. This lack of competition between clot-bound and circulating fibrinogen for the drug creates a higher "gradient" for diffusion of anisoylated drug into the thrombus.

Although APSAC has a number of attractive features, its clinical actions are remarkably similar to those of STK (Table 4.1).

For example, APSAC that is deacylated in the circulation converts plasminogen to plasmin, which in turn causes fibrinogenolysis
(Fig. 4.2). In one clinical study, APSAC caused an 85% decline in
fibrinogen, a 70% fall in plasminogen, and a 99% reduction of
alpha$_2$ antiplasmin; actions which are similar to STK. After 24
hours fibrinogen had returned to 43% of baseline with a return
to normal at 48 hours. Thus, APSAC appears to be as potent
as STK in producing both a systemic lytic state as well as a
hypocoagulable state. Rates of thrombolysis determined by early
angiography have been no different with STK and APSAC. The
major clinical benefit with APSAC appears to be ease of administration since it can be given as a bolus injection.

There is no special toxicity of APSAC when compared with
STK. Because it contains STK it is antigenic. The incidence of
hypotension is slightly higher with APSAC than STK (Table 4.1).

UK

UK is an endogenous protein and can be isolated from human
urine. It has less fibrin affinity than other agents, and uptake of
UK into thrombus is limited (Fig. 4.3). It induces a systemic lytic
state, and the circulating, free plasmin that is formed actively
digests thrombus. Unlike STK, UK is an enzyme which directly
cleaves the light and heavy chain of plasminogen (Fig. 4.6).
It depletes fibrinogen to a lesser degree than STK. There have
been no mortality trials of intravenous UK in MI, and it is not
approved for this use. The drug is commonly given by the intracoronary route in the cardiac catheterization laboratory.

t-PA

t-PA is a naturally occurring protein found both in the circulation
and in thrombus. rt-PA is the same protein which is manufactured
using "genetic engineering" techniques. When it is free in the
circulation, rt-PA is a poor plasminogen activator. When bound
to fibrin, a co-factor, its activity in cleaving the plasminogen
molecule is increased 500-fold (Fig. 4.5). For this reason, it is
much more effective as an activator of fibrin-bound plasminogen
than circulating plasminogen. It is often described as a "clot
specific" or "tissue level" plasminogen activator. Other thrombolytic agents, including STK but not UK, are also more active

when in the presence of fibrin. But with rt-PA, fibrin is required as a co-factor for its action.

There is some fibrinogen depletion during rt-PA therapy because of the huge dose of rt-PA that is given relative to physiologic, circulating levels of native t-PA. Typically, fibrinogen levels fall to 50% of baseline (Table 4.1). rt-PA has a short half-life and is thus infused over 3 hours.

Rethrombosis is more common following rt-PA treatment than with the other thrombolytic agents. There is less fibrinogenolysis, less fibrinogen depletion, and therefore, a lower concentration of fibrin degradation products (which are anticoagulants). For these reasons, full anticoagulant doses of intravenous heparin have been recommended starting 1 hour before the end of rt-PA infusion.

Heparin also directly increases the enzymatic efficiency of rt-PA. By contrast, STK–plasminogen activator complex is not influenced by heparin. This may be important in interpreting trials of heparin as adjunctive therapy for thrombolytic therapy. Some studies of rt-PA have indicated that heparin improves patency rates, but similar trials have not been performed with STK (Chapter 8).

rt-PA may be more effective than other agents in promoting dissolution of older thrombus with cross-linked fibrin. This may explain the higher incidence of intracranial bleeding that has been described with this agent. In the ISIS-3 trials, intracranial bleeding occurred in 0.5% treated with STK, 0.6% with APSAC, and 0.7% with rt-PA; these patients were also treated with subcutaneous heparin. Intracranial bleeding with rt-PA appears to be dose-dependent; it occurred more frequently in early trials using 150 mg rt-PA compared with more recent studies using the currently recommended 100 mg dose. The dose should be lowered further for lighter patients (Chapter 5).

Effectiveness of rt-PA has been found to be greater in trials that used a "front-loaded" dosing regimen. We now use this approach with both rt-PA and STK (Chapter 5).

Comparative trials of thrombolytic agents: which drug should I use?

Thrombolysis may occur 30 minutes earlier with rt-PA than with STK. This 30 minute difference has not had a demonstrable effect in clinical trials comparing the effects of the two drugs on either

Table 4.2 Comparative trials of thrombolytic agents using intravenous therapy

	n	STK	rt-PA	APSAC
Mortality (%)				
GISSI-2	12 490	8.6	9.0	—
ISIS-3	39 913	10.5	10.3	10.6
LVEF (%)				
White	270	58	58	—
CITTS	253	52	53	—
Infarct artery patency (%)[‡]				
ECSG	129	55	70*	—
TIMI-1	290	31	62*	—
PAIMS	171	74	81	—
TEAM2	370	73	—	72
HOGG	128	53	—	55
TEAM3[†]	332	85	—	90
TAPS[†]	433	—	84	70

* Significantly different ($p < 0.05$).
[†] Unpublished data.
[‡] Patency at 90 minutes after starting thrombolytic therapy.

survival or LV function. Recall that these two important clinical endpoints have been favorably influenced by thrombolytic agents when compared with placebo.

Perhaps the most influential study that directly compared drugs was the TIMI-1 trial. In this study, rt-PA was found to be twice as effective as STK in opening occluded arteries when the coronary angiogram was performed 90 minutes after starting therapy (Table 4.1). Delay of thrombolytic therapy for a pretreatment coronary angiogram meant that thrombolytic therapy was given late (4.8 hours after the onset of MI). The more effective 90 minute patency rate with rt-PA was not accompanied by better LV function, an expected finding with therapy begun this late in the course of infarction. Marder and Sherry have analyzed a subset of patients in TIMI-1 who had earlier treatment (within 3 hours of onset of MI). These patients had similar 90 minute patency rates with STK and rt-PA. It is possible that rt-PA is more effective in disrupting "mature" thrombus.

Earlier therapy and earlier restoration of flow should lead to better survival and improved myocardial salvage. On the other hand, an open infarct artery after thrombolytic therapy has also been shown to enhance survival independent of changes in LV function. Speed of action may not be the only factor that determines the clinical benefit of a drug.

Finally, the treatment strategy following thrombolytic therapy may influence LV function and survival endpoints as profoundly as the drugs themselves. Maintaining infarct artery patency with aggressive anticoagulation (both heparin and aspirin), and possibly with revascularization is important and must be considered when evaluating randomized trials. Table 4.2 and Appendix 1 summarize a number of trials comparing thrombolytic agents. With one exception, none has shown that a specific drug provides any special "clinical" benefit.

The sole exception is CITTS which compared effects of STK and rt-PA on LV function. We found no difference in patients with inferior MI. Patients with anterior MI had better anterior, regional wall contractility with rt-PA than they did with STK. A similar study from New Zealand (White, *et al.*, 1989) found no improvement in regional wall motion with rt-PA. Patients in CITTS routinely had early revascularization, and this was avoided in the New Zealand trial. Both of these studies were small, the CITTS results were "suggestive" at best, and we do not believe that this issue is settled. CITTS does indicate a need for larger comparative drug studies using our revascularization strategy after thrombolysis (Chapter 7). It further indicates the need for studies comparing different revascularization techniques. To date, only percutaneous transluminal coronary angioplasty has been studied, and it does not appear to be any more beneficial than medical therapy (TIMI-2). CITTS, which used coronary artery bypass surgery as the initial technique for two-thirds of patients having revascularization, suggests studies which incorporate bypass surgery.

MI is an illness that kills and disables hundreds of thousands of patients yearly. A strong argument can be made for the study of a few tens of thousands in order to identify the most efficacious and cost effective therapeutic approach. A "best" thrombolytic agent for all patients has not been clearly identified based on present studies. It is possible that large trials will find that a specific agent has advantages in a specific clinical setting.

Combination therapy

There have been no trials comparing combinations of thrombolytic agents with placebo. The KAMIT study compared rt-PA plus STK with rt-PA therepy alone. Patients in the combination therapy group were given lower dose rt-PA, 50 mg, in addition to 1.5 ml U STK. All patients had angiography 2–4 hours after receiving thrombolytic therapy. Those in the combination therapy group had significantly higher infarct artery patency. In this trial, patients who had a closed infarct artery at the time of the early angiogram had "rescue" angioplasty. Using this approach, infarct artery patency was achieved in 95% of patients in both treatment groups. The patients who received the combination of rt-PA and STK had less reocclusion and fewer adverse clinical events during the next week. This combination of lower dose rt-PA with conventional dose STK thus appears more effective. It is certainly less expensive than using full dose rt-PA alone. This study found no increase in bleeding risk with combination therapy.

TAMI-2 also reported that abrupt closure of the infarct artery was less common after emergency angioplasty in patients on rt-PA plus UK. The large GUSTO trial will be the first study of combination therapy (STK plus rt-PA 1 mg/kg body weight) that has mortality as the primary endpoint.

A recommendation

Our recent study, CITTS, and all other comparative trials indicate that STK is a suitable choice for patients with inferior MI. The rate of progression of injury in patients with anterior MI may be "faster" than with inferior MI, and rt-PA is a "faster" thrombolytic agent. We recommend rt-PA for patients early in the course of anterior MI. Patients who are treated late in the course of MI, beyond 3–4 hours, may benefit from rt-PA therapy, as it appears to disrupt mature, organized thrombus more rapidly than STK (TIMI-1). APSAC has not been found to be more effective in trials comparing it with STK or rt-PA, but it is easier to administer.

Fibrinogenolysis and bleeding

During the early development of thrombolytic therapy we were concerned that fibrinogen depletion by systemic agents would increase the risk of bleeding. t-PA, which requires fibrin as a co-factor and is thus most active when bound to fibrin, is less active in the circulation and causes less depletion of fibrinogen. For this reason there was hope that it would be a safer agent. That has not been the case. The TIMI-1 trial reported that fibrinogen levels were better maintained with rt-PA than with STK, but the incidence of bleeding was similar. In multiple studies, bleeding has not correlated with the degree of fibrinogen depletion. Instead, bleeding appears to occur at sites of vascular injury, most commonly venipuncture and cardiac catheterization sites.

Finally, rt-PA may be more effective than other agents in dissolving old thrombus. With time, thrombus contracts and increases its density through a process of alpha-chain cross linking. rt-PA may have a greater effect than STK on such mature thrombus. Hemostatic plug is more likely to have older, more mature thrombus than is a freshly occluded artery, and this, theoretically, would increase the bleeding risk with rt-PA. There is concern that this effect of rt-PA on mature thrombus (hemostatic plug) may be responsible for a higher rate of intracranial bleeding.

It has been difficult to separate theoretical risks of fibrinogenolysis from potential benefits. It appears now that the hypocoagulable state produced by fibrinogen depletion is beneficial, as drugs that deplete fibrinogen have lower rates of arterial reocclusion (Table 4.1). Circulating plasmin digests not just fibrinogen but depletes clotting factors V, VIII, and others as well. Fibrin degradation products inhibit platelet activity and other clotting mechanisms. During the 36 hours after thrombolytic therapy, coronary artery lesions are dynamic with thrombus dissolving, then reforming. The hypocoagulable state may improve the chance for maintaining an open artery.

TIMI-1 found reocclusion (using a second angiogram predischarge) in 14% of patients treated with STK and 24% treated with rt-PA. Reocclusion was associated with recurrence of chest pain in just 12–13% of these patients. The implication was that patients with silent reocclusion had "completed" MI, had no viable muscle, and therefore no pain. But a number of recent studies indicate that "silent ischemia" is especially common after thrombolytic therapy. It may be that nerve injury exceeds muscle injury in the infarct zone, and that patients have viable muscle but an inability to transmit ischemic pain through injured nerves. Studies which have relied on recurrence of chest pain to diagnose recurrent ischemia probably underestimated its incidence

(Chapter 7). If further injury occurs with silent reocclusion of infarct arteries, thrombolytic agents and adjunctive therapies that prevent reocclusion are especially important.

Another potential benefit of fibrinogen depletion is reduced viscosity and improved flow in the microcirculation. Fibrinogen is an unusually large molecule, and is asymmetric in shape. It is the most prevalent large molecule in plasma and thus accounts for a substantial proportion of total viscosity. Reduced viscosity has been documented following STK therapy. This may improve coronary microcirculation, although the clinical benefits of this remain unstudied and theoretical.

Cost issues

Table 4.1 reflects our costs for each of the thrombolytic agents. STK (Streptase®) is commonly discounted, as is APSAC (Eminase®). We have been unable to get a discounted price for rt-PA (Activase®). Wholesale costs are misleading. All hospital pharmacies have a markup. We polled 20 hospitals in rural, central Illinois and found that the charge to the patient for administering rt-PA ranges from $1832 to $6237, and that the charge for administering STK ranges from $150 to $979.

The higher cost of any therapy is justified if it results in lower morbidity or mortality. In fact, more effective therapies may reduce the overall cost of care by lowering complication rates. Preventing CHF after acute MI would shorten the length of hospitalization as well as reduce health care costs over the remainder of the patient's life. Topol has reported a series of patients with acute MI treated with rt-PA who had a lower rate of heart failure and could be discharged earlier than others not treated with thrombolytic therapy.

This way of analyzing the effect of therapy on hospital costs can be turned around: perhaps hospital costs or charges can be used as an indicator of the efficacy of a treatment approach. If so, costs might reflect "unmeasurable" clinical benefits of a new treatment such as more rapid recovery of strength or vigor. We have applied such analysis to patients having coronary artery bypass surgery. Multivariate analysis indicated that higher hospital charges after bypass surgery can be most directly attributed to complications (Taylor, et al., 1990). A survey of hospitals in Illinois indicated that low-volume programs tended to have higher hospital charges, raising the possibility that higher hospital charges follow increased

Table 4.3 CITTS: average hospital charge by department (253 patients) (From Taylor, et al., unpublished data)

Total charges[‡]	STK	rt-PA	p
ICU	1970 ± 2177	2071 ± 1739	NS
Laboratory	1393 ± 900	1414 ± 971	NS
Pharmacy[†]	1015 ± 1032	2952 ± 1006	$p < 0.001$
Surgery	5399 ± 2727	6506 ± 2805	$p = 0.03$
Cardiovascular*	4184 ± 2143	4277 ± 2144	NS

* Cardiovascular includes catheterization laboratory charges.
[†] Total charges. Hospital cost for STK was $79 and for rt-PA was $2200. The charge for STK was $186.32 and for rt-PA was $2352.60.

complication rates. Higher morbidity and mortality have been observed in low-volume heart surgery programs.

We have used a similar analysis of cost in the CITTS trial, testing whether costs might indirectly point to a benefit of one of the drugs not immediately, clinically apparent. We prospectively collected hospital cost and charge data and found that the difference in total hospital costs for the STK and rt-PA groups was $1418. This is remarkably close to the difference in cost between the two drugs (Table 4.1). Hospital charges were further analyzed by department. Charges were similar for all these departments with the greatest exception being pharmacy (Table 4.3).

Although CITTS identified improved regional wall motion in a subset of patients with anterior infarction who were treated with rt-PA, this did not translate into a great enough clinical benefit to offset the higher cost of rt-PA.

On the other hand, new therapies are always expensive and actual costs decline with time. This may be the case with rt-PA and APSAC. And we now hear that the price of STK may be raised.

The cost issue is critical at a time when hospitals are struggling financially. We expect that with time, the cost of the agents will become competitive, and drug choices will be based purely on clinical issues.

Selected reading

Anderson JL, Sorensen SG, Moreno FL, et al. Multicenter patency trial of intravenous anistreplase compared with streptokinase in acute myocardial infarction. Circulation 1991;83:126–40.

Anderson JL, *et al*. A randomized trial of APSAC versus t-PA in the United States and Canada: Design, recruitment and demographics for the TEAM-3 investigators (Unpublished data).

Chesebro JH, Knatterud G, Roberts R, *et al*. Thrombolysis in myocardial infarction (TIMI) trial, Phase I: a comparison between intravenous tissue plasminogen activator and intravenous streptokinase. Circulation 1987;76:142–54.

Fears R, Ferres H, Standring R. Evidence for the progressive uptake of anisoylated plasminogen streptokinase activator complex by clots in human plasma *in vitro*. Drugs 1987;33(Suppl 3):51–56.

Ferres H, Hibbs M, Smith RAG. Deacylation studies *in vitro* on anisoylated plasminogen streptokinase activator complex. Drugs 1987;33(Suppl 3):80–82.

Ferres H. Preclinical pharmacological evaluation of anisoylated plasminogen streptokinase activator complex. Drugs 1987;33(Suppl 3): 33–50.

Flores ED, Lange RA, Cigarroa RG, Hillis LD. Southwestern internal medicine conference: Therapy of acute myocardial infarction in the 1990s. Am J Medical Sciences 1990;299:415–24.

GISSI-2. A factorial randomised trial of alteplase versus streptokinase and heparin versus no heparin among 12 490 patients with acute myocardial infarction. Lancet 1990;336:65–71.

Hogg KJ, Gemmill JD, Burns JM, *et al*. Angiographic patency study of anistreplase versus streptokinase in acute myocardial infarction. Lancet 1990;335:254–58.

Grines CL, Nissen SE, Booth DC, *et al*. Kentucky Acute Myocardial Infarction Trial Group. A prospective, randomized trial comparing combination half-dose tissue-type plasminogen activator and streptokinase with full-dose tissue-type plasminogen activator. Circulation 1991;84:540–49.

ISIS-3. Presented at the annual meeting of the American College of Cardiology, Atlanta, Georgia, March 1991.

Magnani B, PAIMS Investigators. Plasminogen activator italian multicenter study (PAIMS): Comparison of intravenous recombinant single-chain human tissue-type plasminogen activator (rt-PA) with intravenous streptokinase in acute myocardial infarction. J Am Coll Cardiol 1989;13:19–26.

Marder VJ, Sherry S. Thrombolytic therapy: Current status. NEJM 1988;318:1512–20.

Neuhaus KL, Tebbe U, Gottwik M, *et al*. Intravenous recombinant tissue plasminogen activator (rt-PA) and urokinase in acute myocardial infarction: Results of the German activator urokinase study (GAUS). J Am Coll Cardiol 1988;12:281–87.

Sherry S. Bleeding complications in thrombolytic therapy. Hosp Pract 1990;25(Suppl 5):1–21.

Sherry S. Pharmacology of anistreplase. Clin Cardiol 1990;13:V3–10.

Sherry S, Marder VJ. Streptokinase and recombinant tissue plasminogen activator (rt-PA) are equally effective in treating acute myocardial infarction. Ann Int Med 1991;114:417–23.

Taylor GJ, Mikell FL, Moses HW, *et al*. Determinants of hospital charges for coronary artery bypass surgery: The economic consequences of postoperative complications. Am J Cardiol 1990;65:309–13.

Taylor GJ, Moses HW, Koester DL, *et al.* Lower hospital charges in patients treated with streptokinase compared with rt-PA (Unpublished data).

Taylor GJ, Miller BD, Engelking N, *et al.* Early signal-averaged ECG predicts late left ventricular ejection fraction (LVEF) after thrombolytic therapy. American Heart Association 1991 (Unpublished data).

Taylor GJ, Moses HW, Becker LC, *et al.* Comparison of intravenous rt-PA and streptokinase therapy for acute ST segment elevation myocardial infarction: Improved regional wall motion in patients with anterior infarction treated with rt-PA (In press).

Topol EJ, Califf RM, George RS, *et al.* Coronary arterial thrombolysis with combined infusion of recombinant tissue-type plasminogen activator and urokinase in patients with acute myocardial infarction. Circulation 1988;77:1100–07.

Topol EJ, Burek K, O'Neill WW. A randomized controlled trial of hospital discharge three days after myocardial infarction in the era of reperfusion. N Engl J Med 1988;318:1083–88.

Verstraete M, Collen D. Pharmacology of thrombolytic drugs. J Am Coll Cardiol 1986;8(B):33–40.

Verstraete M, Bory M, Collen D, *et al.* Randomised trial of intravenous recombinant tissue-type plasminogen activator versus intravenous streptokinase in acute myocardial infarction. Lancet 1985;11:812–17.

White HD, Rivers JT, Maslowski AH, *et al.* Effect of intravenous streptokinase as compared with that of tissue plasminogen activator on left ventricular function after first myocardial infarction. N Engl J Med 1989;320:817–21.

Chapter 5

Initial approach and treatment protocols

You have spent 10 minutes with a patient with chest pain. It is clear that he or she is having acute MI based on history, examination, and ECG. Thrombolytic therapy is indicated, and there are no contraindications. After weighing benefits and risks, you have decided that he or she should be treated. You expect that treatment will be started well within 30 minutes of emergency department admission. That is to say, you are on schedule. You have indicated your choice of drug to the emergency department staff, and they are in the process of mixing it.

Approaching the patient and his or her family

Even in the rush to initiate therapy it is important that the patient and his or her family clearly understand the rationale for treatment and risks. The points we cover include these:

1 you are having a heart attack, and this usually is caused by a blood clot blocking the artery at the site of hardening-of-the-arteries plaque;

2 (STK, rt-PA, APSAC) are drugs that can "dissolve the blood clot" in 80% of patients;

3 treatment with this medicine has been shown to improve heart muscle function and save lives, and for this reason I strongly recommend it;

4 it is best if given early in the course of a heart attack, and that is why we all seem in a hurry;

5 it will not make the heart attack go away but may turn a large heart attack into a smaller one;

6 there is a risk with the medicine, primarily of bleeding, nevertheless, the potential benefits outweigh the risks;

7 you may need other treatment such as heart catheterization, or balloon dilation, or even surgery, but using the clot buster drug *now* is the most important, first step.

Most patients have heard about "clot buster" therapy and need little convincing in this setting of acute MI.

Consent form

Should the patient sign a consent form? We are divided on this issue. It is not mandatory as thrombolytic therapy for acute MI has FDA approval, and we no longer use a consent for "experimental" treatment. The evidence in favor of thrombolytic therapy is so strong that it would be as sensible to have the patient sign a "release" if he or she refuses. On the other hand, the risks of treatment are significant, and 5–12% of patients will die because of the MI despite thrombolytic therapy (Table 1.2). The morbidity and mortality are higher than we see with most surgical operations, including coronary artery bypass surgery. For this reason most of us (at the Prairie Cardiovascular Center) use a consent form. Its goal is to document your discussion of benefits and risks of treatment with the patient and his or her family. Table 5.1 is a consent form that is applicable to treatment with all the thrombolytic agents.

Where to treat

A large number of community hospitals still transfer patients to the CCU before starting thrombolytic agents. This is an egregious error. A delay of 20 minutes should be considered intolerable, and there are few hospitals that can accomplish patient transfer in that period of time. What if the bed is not quite ready? How long will it take for the emergency department nurse to give a report to the CCU staff? Will the CCU nurse wait to mix the drug until the patient arrives? Will all the necessary lines, etc., be in place when the patient arrives in the CCU? How many CCU nurses will be available to "admit" the patient and start drug therapy?

Thrombolytic therapy must be an emergency department procedure, and the emergency department staff must be the hospital's experts in its use (Chapter 10).

Standing orders

Tables 5.2–5.4 are our standing orders for STK (Streptase®), APSAC (Eminase®) and rt-PA (Activase®). We have found that the use of standing orders significantly increases the efficiency in

Table 5.1 Consent for thrombolytic therapy for acute heart attack

Explanation I understand that I am having a heart attack and for this reason am being offered treatment to stop progression of injury to my heart. I understand that the heart attack may be caused by a blood clot which has formed in one of the arteries to my heart. _____ is a drug which can dissolve the blood clot.

I understand that the medicine will be given intravenously. I also understand that the medicine works for 8 of 10 patients.

Risks of the treatment There is a chance I may die from the heart attack despite use of the clot-dissolving medicine. I understand that there is a 5–10% risk of bleeding complications with the medicine. I have been told that my bleeding risks can be serious and include bleeding into the stomach or bowels, bleeding from the kidneys, or bleeding from i.v. or blood-drawing sites. There is a 1–2% risk of bleeding into the brain causing stroke. I realize that any of these bleeding complications could be fatal.

Benefits of the treatment I have been told that the main benefit of treatment is interruption of heart attack so that damage to the heart muscle is limited. Despite the above risks, this treatment improves my chances for surviving the heart attack. It can leave me with a heart that is stronger. This may mean a better chance for recovering exercise ability and possibly improved long-term survival.

Alternative treatments The alternative to this treatment is the routine management of complications of heart attack.

Doctor _____ has discussed the procedure with me and my family and has answered all of our questions.

Subject	Date
Next of kin	Date
Physician	Date
Witness	Date

which patients can be treated. The doctor and nurse do not have to spend time reading the package insert in order to determine how to give the medicine. It works best if there is just *one* set of standing orders for each drug in your institution. Having different standing orders for each physician generates excessive confusion.

Table 5.2 Standing orders — intravenous STK therapy for acute MI

Initial blood work: emergency cardiac panel (this includes *stat* CBC, platelet count, chem. 20, cardiac enzymes, CK-MB fraction, PT, PTT, urinalysis). Do not delay STK for results of urinalysis or blood work

ECG *stat*, I hour after completion of STK and with any change in symptoms

STK drug protocol:
    Dose — 1 500 000 U STK over I hour
    Reconstitution — 1 500 000 U in 45 ml normal saline
    Administration — give 375 000 U (11.25 ml over 5 min)
    Then decrease rate of STK infusion to 37 ml/h to administer remaining
    1 125 000 U (33.75 ml) over 55 min

Two baby aspirin (81 mg) chewed when thrombolytic therapy started and one enteric-coated aspirin (i.e. Ecotrin® 325 mg) p.o. daily as long as patient is not allergic to aspirin

Prophylactic lidocaine, 75 mg bolus intravenously for normal-sized adults. Lidocaine infusion dose to be determined by the attending physician. Do not delay STK infusion for lidocaine!

When the STK infusion bag is empty, infuse 50 ml 0.9% NaCl at the same rate to flush the i.v. line

Administer heparin 5000 U i.v. bolus and begin continuous infusion @ 1000 U/h upon completion of STK

aPTT in 6 hours (call if <70 s)

Routine CCU orders after STK

No arterial sticks including blood gases without checking with physician

Cardiac enzymes 2, 4, 8, 12 hours after *starting* STK

Date: _____   Signed: _____

CBC, complete blood count
PT, prothrombin time; PTT, partial thromboplastin time.

Here are a few observations about the standing orders and how your team should approach these patients:

Initial blood work

Remember that the primary goal is treatment of the patient within 30 minutes of arrival in the emergency department. All efforts must be directed to that end. It makes sense to draw blood work at the time of arrival, but do not wait for laboratory results to decide upon therapy.

Table 5.3 Standing orders — intravenous rt-PA (Activase) therapy for acute MI

Initial blood work: emergency cardiac panel (This includes *stat* CBC, platelet count, chem. 20, cardiac enzymes, CK-MB fraction, PT, PTT, urinalysis). Do not delay rt-PA for results of urinalysis or blood work

ECG *stat*, I hour after starting rt-PA, and with any change in symptoms

Prophylactic lidocaine, 75 mg bolus intravenously for normal-sized adults. Lidocaine infusion rate to be determined by the attending physician. Do not delay rt-PA infusion for lidocaine!

Administer i.v. rt-PA (Activase®) *through separate i.v. line* at the following dose dependent on the patient's weight:

Patient weight ≥65 kg (mix 100 mg rt-PA in 100 ml sterile water):
   10 mg rt-PA bolus i.v. push over 1–2 min (10 ml)
   50 mg i.v. over the first hour (50 ml)
   20 mg i.v. over the second hour (20 ml)
   20 mg i.v. over the third hour (20 ml)

Patient weight <65 kg, total dose of 1.25 mg per kg administered as follows: (mix 1.25 mg rt-PA/kg in 100 ml sterile water)

   10% rt-PA bolus i.v. push over 1–2 min (10 ml)
   50% i.v. over the first hour (50 ml)
   20% i.v. over the second hour (20 ml)
   20% i.v. over the third hour (20 ml)

When the rt-PA infusion bag is empty, infuse 50 ml 0.9% NaCl at the same rate to flush the i.v. line

Administer heparin 5000 U i.v. and begin continuous infusion @ 1000 U/h, I hour after t-PA infusion started

aPTT in 6 hours (call if <70 s)

Two baby aspirin (81 mg) chewed when thrombolytic therapy started and one enteric-coated aspirin (i.e. Ecotrin® 325 mg) p.o. daily as long as patient is not allergic

Routine CCU orders after rt-PA

No arterial sticks including blood gases without checking with physician

Cardiac enzymes 2, 4, 8, 12 hours after starting rt-PA

Date: _____   Signed: _____

One nurse is not enough

Our emergency department protocol calls for at least two nurses to work with these patients with acute MI. In a smaller hospital, you may elect to call a CCU nurse to the emergency department

Table 5.4 Standing orders — intravenous APSAC (Eminase®) therapy for acute MI

Initial blood work: emergency cardiac panel (this includes *stat* CBC, platelet count, chem. 20, cardiac enzymes, CK-MB fraction, PT, PTT, urinalysis). Do not delay Eminase for results of urinalysis or blood work

ECG *stat*, 1 hour after completion of Eminase, and with change in symptoms

Prophylactic lidocaine, 75 mg bolus intravenously for normal-sized adults. Lidocaine drip to be determined by the attending physician. Do not delay Eminase for lidocaine

Eminase drug protocol:
    Dose/reconstitution — 30 U Eminase in 5 ml sterile water
    (*Do not dilute further*)
    Administration — give 30 U (5 ml) Eminase intravenously over 5 min
If Eminase is not administered within 30 min of reconstitution it must be discarded

4 hours after administration of Eminase begin continuous infusion of Heparin @ 1000 U/h

aPTT in 6 hours (call if <70 s)

Two baby aspirin (81 mg) chewed when thrombolytic therapy started and one enteric-coated aspirin (i.e. Ecotrin® 325 mg) p.o. daily as long as patient is not allergic to aspirin

Routine CCU orders after Eminase

No arterial sticks including blood gases without checking with physician

Cardiac enzymes 2, 4, 8, 12 hours after starting Eminase

Date: _____   Signed: _____

to help with chest pain patients during the crucial first 30 minutes. One nurse performs the mechanical tasks (drawing blood, starting i.v. lines, starting oxygen...). The second nurse must focus all attention on starting the thrombolytic drug. All emergency department staff should be trained to perform a 12-lead ECG.

Lidocaine

There has been no study showing that lidocaine improves survival in a setting of thrombolytic therapy. Ventricular ectopy is common during reperfusion, but VF is uncommon as a reperfusion arrhythmia. Nevertheless, earlier studies of prophylactic lidocaine for acute MI (in the absence of thrombolytic therapy) have shown that it reduces the risk of VF. These studies did not show improved survival, as they were conducted in CCUs where prompt defibrillation was available. But fewer patients required cardioversion with prophylactic lidocaine. On the negative side is the risk of lidocaine toxicity which is dose related. Patients who are outside the CCU, especially those who will be transferred from one hospital to another, probably should have prophylactic lidocaine.

Front-loaded dosing

An initial bolus injection of rt-PA has been shown to improve early patency rates. While it has not been studied, we have also routinely used front-loaded dosing with STK. You will recall that there is competition for infused STK between antibodies, circulating plasminogen, and thrombus (Chapter 4). Without front-loading there is a substantial delay before a therapeutic concentration of STK is available at the level of thrombus.

The 86% patency rate we have described in our multiple studies of intravenous STK has been considered high by some observers. Front-loaded dosing with STK may be responsible for this high patency rate. Rothbard and colleagues observed that thrombolysis rarely occurred in patients treated with *intracoronary* STK unless a systemic lytic state had been achieved. Front-loading intravenous STK will produce a lytic state more rapidly.

It takes a fair volume (18–24 ml) to load the i.v. tubing when administering these drugs. Pay attention that drug is being infused and not saline or other line fillers when you start the thrombolytic agent. Front-loading may speed the process of initiating drug infusion. For the same reasons, flushing the i.v. lines is important at the end of infusion with both STK and rt-PA so that all drug is infused. i.v. tubing with in-line filters should not be used; the filters have been shown to decrease efficacy with rt-PA, and we do not use filtered lines with any of these agents.

Drug reconstitution

This is straight-forward with all of the drugs (Tables 5.2–5.4). The standard dose of STK is 1 500 000 iu for all patients. The dose of rt-PA is adjusted if the patient weighs <65 kg. Both APSAC and rt-PA are mixed in sterile water. APSAC must be given within 30 minutes of mixing it or it must be discarded.

Heparin

Heparin is started at the end of the STK infusion, 1 hour before the end of the rt-PA infusion and 4–6 hours after giving APSAC.

Aspirin

This will be discussed in Chapter 8 with other forms of adjunctive therapy. But aspirin at the time of initial presentation is so clearly beneficial that we have included it in our standing orders. Other adjunctive therapies (beta blockers, nitrates, etc.) must be added by the physician. We use the same dose of aspirin that was used in the ISIS-2 trial (Appendix 1). In this study, 160 mg aspirin was chewed in order to achieve a rapid blood level. Chewing two baby aspirin is easy for most patients.

Routine CCU orders

These are used after administration of the thrombolytic agent. Once you have given the thrombolytic agent, the monitoring protocol is no different than standard practice. The only difference is more frequent CK measurements in the first 12 hours in order to detect early CK washout. Treatment of arrhythmias, LV failure, pulmonary congestion, and other complications of infarction are unaffected by thrombolytic agents.

Arterial sticks

There is one important exception to this statement about routine care and that is arterial sticks for blood gas analysis. "Routine" blood gas draws have caused some of the worst complications of thrombolytic therapy we have seen. The brachial artery will continue to bleed following puncture when thrombolytic agents are on board. The thrombolytic drugs do work, and it is almost impossible to form hemostatic plug at an arterial puncture site. The patient may lose 2–3 units of blood into the antecubital fossa, and it is not a pretty sight. It is for this reason that we have specifically proscribed arterial sticks on standing orders. The physician may forget, and this order prompts the nurse to remind him. Our nurses routinely place a sign at the head of the bed that states "No Arterial Sticks!"

It is rare that arterial blood gases are needed for patients with acute MI. If you are concerned about possible respiratory failure, particularly for patients with advanced obstructive lung disease or severe heart failure, order blood gases, then be prepared to apply pressure to the arterial puncture site long term. (As Sherry has said, use a sandbag, then have someone on hand to stand on the sandbag.)

If excessive bleeding seems likely, surgical repair of the arterial puncture site may be needed.

Selected reading

Korsmeyer C, Midden A, Taylor GJ. The nurse's role in thrombolytic therapy for acute MI. Critical Care Nurse 1987;7:22–30.

Taylor GJ, Mikell FL, Koester DL, *et al*. CITTS. Comparison of intravenous tissue plasminogen activator (rt-PA) and streptokinase therapy for acute ST-segment elevation myocardial infarction: Improved regional wall motion in patients with anterior infarction treated with rt-PA. The Central Illinois Thrombolytic Therapy Study (CITTS) (Unpublished data).

Taylor GJ, Song A, Moses HW, *et al*. The primary care physician and thrombolytic therapy for acute myocardial infarction: Comparison of intravenous streptokinase in community hospitals and the tertiary referral center. J Am Board Fam Pract 1990;3:1–6.

Rothbard RL, Fitzpatrick PG, Francis CW, *et al*. Relationship of the lytic state to successful reperfusion with stand- and low-dose intracoronary streptokinase. Circulation 1985;71:562–70.

Chapter 6

Clinical management during the first 36 hours after thrombolytic therapy

Bedside assessment of early reperfusion

Clinical response

Patients respond to thrombolytic therapy with one of three clinical patterns. The first is the easiest to identify, but occurs in less than half of the patients treated. The patient experiences a sudden relief of chest pain, and ST segments return to baseline. There may be reperfusion ventricular ectopy, and accelerated idioventricular rhythm (AIVR) commonly follows reperfusion (Fig. 6.1). These arrhythmias are short-lived, and VT or VF are rare.

At the other extreme is the patient who has persistent chest pain and unrelieved ST segment elevation. Reperfusion is less likely with this pattern, but even continued pain does not preclude opening of the infarct artery. The patient's symptoms and ECG response are not reliable guides.

An intermediate response is common. The patient may have some improvement in the ECG and some reduction in chest discomfort, but the result is not a dramatic one. Many patients with this intermediate response have an open infarct artery and salvage of myocardium. Commonly, they will have an element of discomfort that lasts for hours, but it is not as severe as the initial pain.

Q waves

Regardless of clinical response, evolution of Q waves on the ECG usually occurs after thrombolysis. With reperfusion, Q waves may develop in minutes (Fig. 3.2). The Q wave loses much of its significance in patients treated with thrombolytic therapy. When acute infarction is not treated with thrombolytic therapy, Q waves indicate transmural scar, a "completed" infarction. Angiography

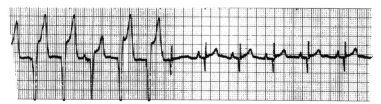

Fig. 6.1 AIVR: a 48-year-old patient with anterior MI treated 2 hours after onset of pain. Shortly after resolution of chest pain and ST segment elevation he developed this ventricular rhythm with a rate of 90–100 beats/minute. This "slow VT" pattern is common with reperfusion. It is considered an "automatic" rather than "re-entrant" rhythm.

Table 6.1 Significance of Q waves after thrombolytic therapy for acute MI (From Mikell, et al.)

	Open infarct artery	Closed infarct artery
Number patient	100	31
Percentage with Q waves	88	87
Percentage with normal regional wall motion	42	15*
LVEF[†] (%)	53	46*

* $p < 0.05$.
[†] RNA 7–10 days after MI.

or other LV imaging studies show a region of akinesis (absent contractility) in the region indicated by the Q wave.

But after thrombolytic therapy, we and others have shown that patients who develop Q waves frequently have recovery of contractility in the infarct zone (Table 6.1). Patients with an open infarct artery after thrombolytic therapy developed Q waves as frequently as those with a closed infarct artery, but they had better regional and global LV contractility. With reperfusion therapy, the Q wave is no longer a reliable indicator of "completed" infarction.

As an aside, we have also found this to be the case for many who have heart surgery and develop Q waves on the postoperative ECG. The mechanism is the same. There is transient ischemia during surgery, then reperfusion and rapid evolution of Q waves despite maintained contractility in the "infarct zone" (Taylor, *et al.*, 1988).

In this same vein, consider the concept of infarct "extension." This has been observed in roughly 10% of patients with MI who develop Q waves. After 1–5 symptom-free days following MI, there is a recurrence of pain, ST segment changes, and CK elevation. Older textbooks had elaborate diagrams of a ring of peri-infarction muscle with presumed marginal blood flow. Somehow this was precipitously lost at the time of infarct "extension," but there was never an explanation for how this peri-infarction zone was precipitously injured. What vessel closed? A better explanation is that this 10% of patients with MI had spontaneous thrombolysis early in the course of infarction and developed Q waves with early reperfusion. The unstable and tightly stenosed artery reoccluded days later resulting in "completion" rather than "extension" of the MI.

We recently had a doctor call about a patient who was treated with thrombolytic therapy, "but it didn't work because he developed Q waves and the enzymes went up." He called when the patient "extended the infarct" days later.

The important message about clinical assessment of thrombolytic therapy is that clinical response and appearance of the ECG are unreliable indicators of clinical efficacy.

Cardiac enzymes

Most patients also have elevation of CK. In fact, when the infarct artery opens early, there is prompt "wash-out" of CK from the infarct zone resulting in early appearance of CK in the circulation, a shorter time to peak CK, and a higher CK spike. Before thrombolytic therapy we measured cardiac enzymes at 4–6 hour intervals during the course of infarction, and we expected to see CK elevation 12 hours after the onset of MI. When treating patients after thrombolytic therapy we measure CK and CK-MB at 2, 4, 8, and 12 hours after treatment in order to detect much earlier CK appearance and thus identify patients with early reperfusion. As an example, the CITTS trial found that 60% of patients had substantial CK elevation (at least twice normal) 2 hours after receiving thrombolytic therapy.

Cardiac arrhythmias

A variety of cardiac rhythm disturbances may occur after thrombolytic therapy for acute MI (Table 6.2). Most are caused by infarction, not reperfusion. Recognition and treatment of arrhythmias are not changed by thrombolytic therapy. This brief survey will emphasize any contribution of reperfusion to the genesis or correction of the arrhythmia.

Table 6.2 Cardiac rhythms commonly observed in the first 36 hours following MI

Rhythm (incidence)	Associated conditions	Treatment and treatment goals
NSR	—	Consider prophylactic lidocaine if the patient is away from the CCU
Isolated VPBs, pairs, short salvos (~50%)	No correlation with LV function	Lidocaine, procainamide; check magnesium and potassium
AIVR (15–30%)	Common with reperfusion, usually temporary	No specific therapy needed; check magnesium and potassium
VT-VF (20%)	No correlation with LV function	DC cardioversion, lidocaine, procainamide, bretylium. Check magnesium and potassium
Sinus tachycardia (40%)	Poor LV function	Treat underlying heart failure
Atrial fibrillation, flutter (15%)	Poor LV function	Control rate with digoxin, verapamil, beta blockers (if no contraindication). Control heart failure. Cardioversion or rapid atrial pacing if hemodynamically unstable
Paroxysmal supraventricular tachycardia (5%)	Poor LV function, excessive sympathetic tone	Vagal maneuvers, verapamil, digoxin, beta blockers, cardioversion, or rapid atrial pacing. Take care not to precipitate heart failure

Table 6.2 *Continued*

Rhythm (incidence)	Associated conditions	Treatment and treatment goals
Sinus bradycardia (25%)	Inferior MI	Treat only if there is hemodynamic compromise. Atropine, pacemaker
AV block narrow QRS (20%)	Inferior MI	Treat only if there is hemodynamic compromise. Atropine or temporary pacemaker
AV block wide QRS (rare)	Inferior or anterior MI	Temporary pacemaker

NSR, normal sinus rhythm.

Reperfusion arrhythmias

Patients commonly have ventricular premature beats (VPBs), short bursts of VT, and occasionally AIVR at the time of reperfusion after thrombolytic therapy. AIVR occurs commonly enough with reperfusion that it is considered a reliable marker of thrombolysis. In a small percentage of patients, these arrhythmias may be dangerous. However, the large, placebo-controlled trials (GISSI-1, ISIS-2, Appendix 1) have shown no difference in the incidence of VF in patients treated with STK and placebo (Table 6.3). In our large series of patients treated in community hospitals, nonsustained VT occurred in 25%, and only 3% of our patients required DC cardioversion for either VT or VF. All were on prophylactic lidocaine.

The mechanisms of reperfusion and ischemic arrhythmias may be different. Ligating a coronary artery in experimental animals causes *prolongation* of the refractory period in the ischemic zone as well as slowed conduction. Most of the arrhythmias arise from the border zone, and are related to heterogeneity of refractoriness between ischemic and normal areas. VF threshold falls during the first day, but it subsequently normalizes. This may be why VF after MI is most common in the first day.

Reperfusion arrhythmias are different. Temporarily ligating a coronary artery in experimental animals causes a fall in fibrilla-

Table 6.3 Incidence of VF in placebo-controlled trials of thrombolytic therapy

Trial (drug)	VF (%)	
	Thrombolytic therapy	Placebo
GISSI-1 (STK)	388/5860 (6.6)	439/5852 (7.5)
ISIS-2 (STK)	370/8490 (4.4)	425/8491 (5.0)
ECSG (rt-PA)	2/64 (3.1)	3/65 (4.6)
ASSET (rt-PA)	94/2516 (3.7)	116/2495 (4.6)
ISAM (STK)	37/859 (4.3)	46/882 (5.2)
White (STK)	1/107 (0.9)	1/112 (0.9)

tion threshold, but also *shortening* of the refractory period and "fractionation" of the action potential in the ischemic zone. Unlike ischemia, there are no "late potentials," or persistent electrical activity seen at the end of the QRS complex. It has been suggested that the mechanism of ventricular ectopy with reperfusion involves increased automaticity rather than re-entry (Fig. 6.2). AIVR, which is common after reperfusion, is considered an automatic rather than a re-entrant arrhythmia.

It is easy to experimentally induce reperfusion VF. But, as a clinical entity, reperfusion VF may be rare, probably because of the duration of ischemia before reperfusion. In experimental animals the duration of ischemia is critical, with severe arrhythmias occurring when ischemia is released just before there is cell death in the subendocardium. The arrhythmias occur only when there is reversible cellular injury. If ischemia is long enough to cause cell death, reperfusion arrhythmias are uncommon, and this may be the case for most patients with MI and thrombolytic therapy. This is consistent with the clinical observation that serious reperfusion arrhythmias are more common in patients who have early rather than late reperfusion. Mathey, *et al.*, 1981 described patients treated with intracoronary STK 1.4 hours after

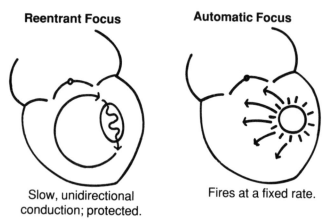

Reentrant Focus

Automatic Focus

Slow, unidirectional
conduction; protected.

Fires at a fixed rate.

Fig. 6.2 Mechanisms for VT. Re-entry occurs when there is a region of myocardium that has slow, unidirectional conduction and that is "insulated" from surrounding tissue. By the time current exits the re-entrant focus, the ventricle has repolarized and is ready for stimulation. Current passes through the remainder of the ventricle, re-enters the protected focus and a circuit is established with repetitive firing. Automatic focus: an automatic focus fires spontaneously at a fixed rate, and works like a fixed rate pacemaker. If the normal heart rate is faster than the rate of the automatic focus, ectopy will not be seen. But if the heart rate falls below that of the automatic focus the patient will have an AIVR (Fig. 6.1).

Table 6.4 Influence of corrected QT interval (QTc) on ventricular arrhythmia after acute MI (From Taylor, et al., 1981. QT corrected for heart rate using Bazett's formula: $QTc = QT\sqrt{R\text{-}R}$)

	QTc (s)			
	Admission	Day 2	Day 3	Day 5
Patients with VT	0.52	0.50	0.49	0.47
Patients without ventricular ectopy	0.46	0.47	0.47	0.46
	$p < 0.001$	$p < 0.004$	NS	NS

onset of pain; VT or VF occurred in 17%. Studies of patients treated more than 5 hours from onset of pain reported that these arrhythmias were less common. If your patient comes in early after the onset of MI and is treated promptly, reperfusion, ventricular ectopy and VF may occur. Fortunately, reperfusion VF is rarely fatal.

Although malignant reperfusion arrhythmias are probably rare in patients with acute MI receiving thrombolytic therapy, they may play a role in sudden death syndrome. Most patients with sudden death do not have MI. An occluded coronary artery is found at autopsy in only 30% of patients with sudden death syndrome compared with 90% or more in patients with Q wave MI. Patients with sudden death syndrome often have "contraction band necrosis" of myocardium, a pathological finding which indicates transient ischemia with reperfusion. One mechanism of sudden death may be identical to the experimental model of transient coronary artery occlusion, release of ischemia before there is cell death, and reperfusion VT or VF.

Ventricular arrhythmias and acute MI

Although reperfusion ventricular ectopy does occur, most of the malignant ventricular arrhythmias we treat after thrombolytic therapy are related to ischemia and infarction, and not to reperfusion. As noted above, acute ischemia causes heterogeneity in conduction velocity and refractory periods. This heterogeneity sets the stage for re-entrant arrhythmias which are common in the 24 hours after coronary thrombosis (Fig. 6.2). This "electrical phenomenon" is unrelated to size of the infarction. Patients who have VT or VF in the first day after MI have predischarge LVEF that is no lower than patients who did not have the early arrhythmia. Thus, the early arrhythmia does not adversely influence late prognosis (as long as the arrhythmia is treated successfully).

Heterogeneous conduction and repolarization patterns at the time of acute ischemia may produce prolongation of the QT interval. We have found that patients who have QT prolongation early in the course of acute MI are more likely to have VT (Table 6.4). An interaction of acute ischemia with other conditions that lengthen the QT interval may increase the risk of early ventricular arrhythmias. Patients with depressed serum potassium and magnesium have prolonged QT intervals, and these electrolyte abnormalities may be induced by diuretic therapy. It is especially important to measure these electrolytes in patients with acute infarction as replacement may help prevent arrhythmias. Correction of the magnesium and potassium deficits may save the patient with a resistant arrhythmia.

Complex ventricular ectopy which occurs in the *late* hospital phase, 6–8 days after MI, is different than early ventricular ectopy. The late arrhythmia appears to be closely associated with large infarction and depressed LV function. If you find complex late ventricular arrhythmias you may expect to see low ejection fraction, and if you identify low ejection fraction, you may expect the 24 hour monitor to show complex arrhythmias.

The treatment of complex late hospital ventricular ectopy, including nonsustained VT, has been radically altered by the CAST trial. In this study patients with complex ectopy were randomly treated with antiarrhythmic drug therapy or placebo. The two study drugs, flecainide and encainide, were found to double the rate of sudden death when compared with placebo. We no longer treat all patients who have late ectopy with anti-arrhythmic drugs. Instead, we are careful to normalize serum potassium and magnesium, and we optimize heart failure therapy when LV function is depressed. If the patient has recurrent VT and especially sustained VT, we then recommend directed therapy using electrophysiologic testing.

In our experience, another common cause of VT or fibrillation after thrombolytic therapy is reocclusion of the infarct artery and recurrence of ischemia. We recently performed angioplasty on a 54-year-old man 2 days following thrombolytic therapy. During a 3 minute balloon occlusion of the right coronary artery, he developed no chest pain but did have ST segment elevation and a small rise in pulmonary wedge pressure (apparently "silent ischemia"). He developed VT after 3 minutes of balloon induced ischemia. Silent ischemia appears common after thrombolytic therapy. An increase in ventricular ectopy may alert you to infarct artery reocclusion prompting important changes in management. At the least, you should repeat the ECG and possibly cardiac enzymes.

An occasional patient will have malignant ventricular arrhythmias with recurrent VT or VF resistant to drug therapy and requiring repeated DC cardioversion. Ventricular ectopy that is this severe probably is unrelated to thrombolysis and reperfusion. Instead, such patients usually have a large area of injury and depressed LV function, often with heart failure or cardiogenic shock.

In our recent trial of 253 patients treated early with thrombolytic agents (CITTS), 42 patients had LVEF <30% at cardiac

Table 6.5 Antiarrhythmic drugs often needed during the first 36 hours after MI

	Dose	
Drugs	Loading (i.v.)	Maintenance
Lidocaine*	1–3 mg/kg over 3 min	1–3 mg/min i.v.
Procainamide	6–13 mg/kg over 15–20 min	2–6 mg/min i.v. or 350–1000 mg p.o. q 3–6 h
Bretylium[†]	5–10 mg/kg over 5–10 min	0.5–2 mg/min i.v.
Amiodarone[‡]	5–10 mg/kg over 20–30 min	1 g/24 h p.o.
Propranolol§	0.25–0.05 mg, q 5 min, total dose ≤0.15–0.20 mg/kg	10–200 mg p.o. q 6–8 h
Digoxin	0.75–1.0 mg in divided doses	0.125–0.25 mg p.o. daily
Verapamil§	5–10 mg over 1–2 min	0.005 mg/kg per min i.v. or 80–120 mg p.o. q 8 h
Propafenone	1–2 mg/kg	150–300 mg p.o. q 8–12 h
Magnesium	1 g MgSO₄ q 1 h ×4 doses	Magnesium gluconate 500 mg p.o. q 8 h

p.o., oral.

* A single bolus injection of lidocaine followed by maintenance infusion may result in subtherapeutic levels 1–2 hours later. A second bolus of 1/2 mg per kg at that time re-establishes therapeutic levels without changing the maintenance infusion rate. Any time the infusion rate is increased it should be accompanied by a bolus injection. The dose must be lowered in patients with heart failure or shock. Check the lidocaine level 3–5 hours after starting therapy and adjust to a therapeutic concentration of 1–5 µg/ml.

[†] Bretylium is the only antiarrhythmic drug that may convert VF. With recurrent VF we move to this drug promptly.

[‡] Intravenous amiodarone is experimental at this time.

§ May depress LV function. Both metoprolol and atenolol may also be given intravenously; we more commonly use i.v. propranolol for atrial tachyarrhythmias.

catheterization or cardiogenic shock, and one of them died with VF. No patient died with VF in the absence of LV failure.

The treatment of these complex arrhythmias is no different for patients with thrombolytic therapy than it is for others with MI. If lidocaine fails to control the arrhythmia we treat patients with either intravenous procainamide or bretylium tosylate (Table 6.5).

An important management issue at the time of thrombolytic therapy is the prophylactic use of lidocaine for patients without ventricular arrhythmias. There have been no studies indicating a clear benefit with lidocaine therapy for patients having thrombolytic therapy; it has not been shown to reduce incidence of serious reperfusion arrhythmias. Prophylactic lidocaine has been studied in patients with MI not having thrombolytic therapy. Survival was not altered by lidocaine therapy, as these studies were done in the CCU where VF was successfully treated with DC cardioversion. On the other hand, prophylactic lidocaine did lower the incidence of VF and reduce the need for DC cardioversion. This experience would indicate that prophylactic lidocaine may be especially useful for patients who are away from the CCU. For example, patients who are being transferred from one hospital to another or patients who have not yet reached the hospital may benefit from prophylactic lidocaine. Most patients who are sent to us from surrounding hospitals during the 36 hours after thrombolytic therapy are treated with lidocaine during transfer.

Atrial tachyarrhythmias

A variety of atrial arrhythmias may occur early after acute MI including paroxysmal supraventricular tachycardia, atrial fibrillation or flutter and sinus tachycardia (Table 6.2). Unlike early ventricular arrhythmias, atrial tachyarrhythmias early in the course of MI are most common in patients with large infarction. This is true of sinus tachycardia as well as the other atrial arrhythmias. Such patients are more likely to have CHF while in hospital and depressed LVEF at the time of discharge. The atrial arrhythmias, including sinus tachycardia, thus indicate a worse prognosis.

The first goal in treatment of atrial arrhythmias is control of ventricular rate (Table 6.5). This is rarely necessary with sinus tachycardia at a rate <130 beats/minute. It would make no sense to try to suppress sinus tachycardia with drugs that would also depress LV function when the rhythm itself occurs as compensation for poor LV function. Do not make the mistake of trying to lower heart rate in patients with sinus tachycardia with verapamil or beta blockers as this may precipitate heart failure.

Other atrial tachyarrhythmias may require heart rate lowering therapy when ventricular rates are above 130 beats/minute. Digoxin, verapamil, and beta blockers all work, and digoxin is the only one of these therapies that does not depress the left ventricle. Digoxin would be our first choice for patients with possible

LV failure. After heart rate has been controlled using drugs that block conduction in the AV node, cardioversion can be attempted with quinidine or intravenous procainamide. If the atrial arrhythmia is paroxysmal, intravenous procainamide would be our first choice during the first 36 hours after MI to prevent reoccurrence. Propafenone has also been effective with paroxysmal atrial arrhythmias (Table 6.5). When the atrial tachyarrhythmia causes hypotension or apparent hemodynamic collapse, do not hesitate to use synchronized DC cardioversion.

Bradyarrhythmias

Bradyarrhythmias complicating acute infarction tend to improve with reperfusion. Inferior MI is often complicated by sinus bradycardia, first degree AV block, the Wenckebach phenomenon, and even complete heart block (Fig. 6.3). The artery to the AV node originates from the distal right coronary artery and acute occlusion slows conduction in the AV node. With reperfusion, AV nodal conduction improves and there is prompt improvement in heart block. The AV node has both parasympathetic and sympathetic innervation. Both atropine and isoproterenol are generally effective in raising heart rate. Isoproterenol may exacerbate ventricular arrhythmias, and atropine would be our first choice of agents to increase heart rate. We generally reserve the use of atropine for patients with bradycardia who also have a fall in blood pressure or cardiac output. Temporary transvenous pacemaker therapy may be needed. Since reperfusion helps heart block, a need for temporary pacing is less common when patients receive thrombolytic therapy.

A small number of patients with heart block after acute infarction have ischemia below the AV node. There is ischemic injury or dysfunction of the His-Purkinje system running through the interventricular septum. Anterior infarction is the most common cause of septal ischemia and infranodal block (Fig. 6.3). The arrhythmia is characterized by a wide QRS complex with a BBB conduction pattern, Mobitz II or complete heart block, and more profound bradycardia with a ventricular rate below 30 beats/minute. The "takeover" pacemaker deep within the ventricular myocardium is less responsive to atropine and catecholamines, and temporary pacing is essential. Prognosis is poor, not just because of the heart block, but because of the size of the infarction. Many of these patients die with cardiogenic shock. A

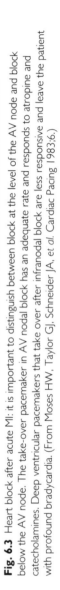

Location of Heart Block	Classification and ECG Appearance	QRS Duration	Origin of Escape Rythm with Complete Heart Block	Prognosis	MI Location	Incidence
AV Node Block (SAN BLOCK AVN)	1. First degree AV Block PR≥0.22 sec 2. Wenckebach, Mobitz 1, Block P P P P 3. Complete heart block P P P P P	Normal (≤0.12 sec) rarely has associated bundle branch block	AV Node Heart rate rate≥40 beats/min	Good (Usually spontaneous recovery)	Inferior MI (Right coronary artery supplies the AV node in 85%)	Common
Infranodal Block (SAN BLOCK AVN)	1. Mobitz II P P P P 2. Complete Heart Block P P P P P	Wide (≥0.12 sec)	Ventricular Conduction System Usually Heart rate < 20 beats/min	Poor (Large MI, heart failure)	Anterior MI (Septal ischemia)	Rare

Fig. 6.3 Heart block after acute MI: it is important to distinguish between block at the level of the AV node and block below the AV node. The take-over pacemaker in AV nodal block has an adequate rate and responds to atropine and catecholamines. Deep ventricular pacemakers that take over after infranodal block are less responsive and leave the patient with profound bradycardia. (From Moses HW, Taylor GJ, Schneider JA, et al. Cardiac Pacing 1983;6.)

temporary pacemaker should be inserted promptly in patients with heart block and wide QRS complex in a setting of acute MI. Many of them will require permanent pacemaker therapy. Like AV nodal block, infranodal heart block may improve with thrombolytic therapy and reperfusion.

In recent years we have placed fewer transvenous temporary pacemakers because of the availability of the transcutaneous pacemaker. "Prophylactic" transvenous pacing is often avoided. The transcutaneous pacemaker is especially helpful in treating patients after thrombolytic therapy since it does not require venous access, fluoroscopy, or experience with right heart catheterization.

Another mechanism of bradyarrhythmia after reperfusion is the Bezold–Jarish reflex. It is attributed to stimulation of chemoreceptors in the left ventricle which in turn increase vagal tone producing bradycardia and/or hypotension. It responds to atropine and volume infusion, and is usually short-lived.

CHF

The clinical diagnosis of LV failure usually is straight forward. The patient has pulmonary rales on physical examination, possibly an S_3 gallop, and pulmonary congestion on the chest X-ray. With worsening LV failure, hypotension may occur, but a common dilemma is our inability to distinguish volume overload from dehydration in patients after acute MI. Low blood pressure and low urinary output may be encountered in a patient who does not have pulmonary congestion. Does he or she need catacholamine therapy or a fluid' challenge? Cardiology consultation and placement of a pulmonary artery catheter may be helpful.

Evaluation of LV function in patients with acute MI

The balloon floatation pulmonary artery catheter is a straightforward device, and I digress to describe it briefly as noncardiologists often consider it complex and esoteric (Fig. 6.4). It is used to determine LV diastolic or "filling" pressure, and diastolic pressure is roughly proportional to the diastolic volume. Adequate diastolic volume in the left ventricle is necessary for the ventricle to generate adequate force of contraction and stroke volume (the Starling mechanism, Figs 6.5, 6.6). Simply put, if the

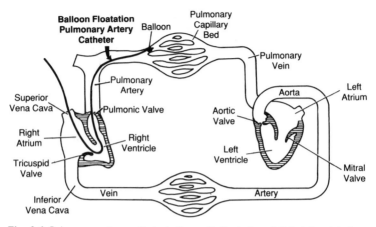

Fig. 6.4 Pulmonary artery catheterization: with the balloon inflated, "wedging" the catheter into a pulmonary artery branch, there is an open channel from the end of the catheter through the pulmonary capillary bed, pulmonary veins, and left atrium to the left ventricle. This allows measurement of LV diastolic pressure, the x axis of the LV function curve.

pump, or left ventricle, does not have enough fluid in it at the beginning of the stroke, stroke output will be low.

Direct measurement of LV diastolic pressure requires arterial catheterization and passage of the catheter across the aortic valve (Fig. 6.4). While this is routinely done in the cardiac catheterization laboratory, it is not a suitable technique for monitoring LV function in the CCU. LV diastolic pressure can be monitored by measuring the occluded pulmonary artery pressure, or "pulmonary wedge pressure." During diastole, the mitral valve is open, and there is no physical structure separating the left ventricle, left atrium, pulmonary vein, pulmonary capillary bed, and pulmonary artery (Fig. 6.4). By "wedging" the catheter into the pulmonary artery with an inflated balloon, there is an open channel from the tip of the pulmonary artery catheter to the left ventricle. The Swan Ganz catheter thus measures LV diastolic pressure. This pulmonary wedge pressure, or LV "filling pressure" is the x axis of the LV function curve (Figs 6.5, 6.6).

Normal LV filling pressure is 8–10 mmHg. Patients who have had MI require LV filling pressure 14–18 mmHg to generate adequate cardiac output, and pressure that is below 10–12 mmHg may indicate volume depletion. When LV filling pressure is above 25 mmHg, hydrostatic pressure in the pulmonary capillary bed exceeds plasma oncotic pressure (which tends to keep fluid in the vascular space), and fluid leaks into the interstitial space causing pulmonary edema.

Treatment of heart failure

Patients who develop pulmonary rales (Killip class II) or pulmonary edema (Killip class III) following acute MI have worse prognosis. Killip described 38% in-hospital mortality rates for those with pulmonary edema (Table 2.2). Causes of death include resistant ventricular arrhythmias as well as heart failure. Atrial arrhythmias are more common in patients with CHF, and they are easier to control after heart failure has been treated. Pharmacologic therapy of heart failure after MI includes the following.

Diuretics
You must relieve pulmonary congestion. We most commonly use intravenous furosemide (Lasix®), a powerful, short-acting diuretic (Table 6.6). Furosemide has been shown to lower LV filling pressure (pulmonary capillary wedge pressure) independent of its diuretic effect; this is especially useful for patients with pulmonary edema. Those who have not been previously treated with diuretics are given 20 mg furosemide intravenously. If this does not elicit prompt diuretic response, twice this dose is given 20–30 minutes later, and the dose is doubled at 30 minute intervals until diuresis is induced. Remember that the duration of action of furosemide is brief. For patients with severe pulmonary congestion, monitor urine output carefully and repeat the effective furosemide dose when urine output falls below 150 ml/hour. Relief of pulmonary congestion is critical, and the only alternatives to diuretics are phlebotomy, ultrafiltration, or hemodialysis.

Diuretics do not improve cardiac function. LV filling pressure or pulmonary capillary wedge pressure falls and congestion is relieved, but cardiac output, stroke work index, or other indices of LV function are worse, not better (Fig. 6.5). In addition to relieving pulmonary congestion you must also do something to improve cardiac output.

Afterload reduction therapy
Reducing peripheral vascular resistance, or cardiac afterload, increases cardiac output at any given level of LV filling pressure

Table 6.6 Treatment of pulmonary congestion/edema and cardiogenic shock

Drugs	Initial dose	Maintenance dose	Onset of action	Duration of action	Comments
Furosemide (Lasix)	20–80 mg i.v.	Titrate to effect	<5 min	2–4 hours	Low initial dose if no prior exposure to furosemide; double dose q 20–30 min until diuresis is achieved
Afterload reduction, intravenous therapy					
Nitroglycerin	10 μ/min	10–150 μg/min	<5 min	~30 min	Do not push systolic pressure <100 mmHg
Catecholamines, intravenous therapy					
Dopamine	2 μg/kg per min	2–10 μg/kg per min	<2 min	<5 min	At low dose it increases renal blood flow and may help with diuresis
Dobutamine	2 μg/kg per min	2–10 μg/kg per min	<2 min	<5 min	A pure inotropic agent, less apt to provoke ectopy
Dopamine plus dobutamine	—	Each at 7.5 μg/kg per min i.v.	—	—	An especially effective combination when higher dose therapy is needed to maintain blood pressure
IABP	—	—	Immediate	—	The most effective "afterload reducer"; best results with an open infarct artery*

* The chance of saving the patient with IABP therapy alone, without reperfusion therapy, is quite poor. A common experience is to have a patient "stuck" on IABP with little chance for survival.

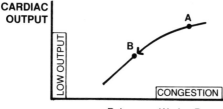

Fig. 6.5 LV function curve illustrating diuretic therapy for heart failure: the patient begins at point A with a high pulmonary wedge pressure (usually above 25 mmHg) and frank pulmonary congestion. Diuresis is critical to relieve pulmonary edema. Removing fluid lowers LV volume and reduces wedge pressure. Congestion is relieved, but cardiac output also is lower (point B). Low cardiac output, in turn, means reduced renal perfusion and a tendency to retain salt and water.

(Fig. 6.6). During acute MI, intravenous nitroglycerin is a good afterload reducer (Table 6.6). It is safe and it is easy to use. In addition to reducing afterload, nitroglycerin reduces preload which helps pulmonary congestion. These actions may limit the size of MI. Nitroglycerin also dilates collateral vessels and may improve flow to areas that have borderline ischemia (again reducing infarct size). Finally, intravenous nitroglycerin has a short half-life, and its effects dissipate quickly if there are problems (i.e. severe hypotension). Afterload reduction therapy should be considered especially for patients with hypertension. It can be used in patients with systolic blood pressures of 90–110 mmHg, but with caution.

How can you give a drug which lowers peripheral vascular resistance to a patient who already has borderline hypotension? The answer is in the hydraulics equation:

pressure = resistance × flow.

When resistance is lowered, flow increases, and pressure is unchanged. If there is overshoot and resistance is lowered by an amount that cannot be offset by an increase in flow, then hypotension will result. In patients with borderline low blood pressure the dose of intravenous nitroglycerin has to be titrated carefully. We usually start with 5–10 μg/minute and gradually raise the dose until blood pressure begins to fall. For patients with borderline hypotension it is unusual that more than 20–30 μg/minute can be tolerated. But in patients who are hypertensive, it is

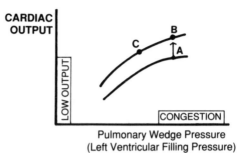

Fig. 6.6 Afterload reduction and inotropic therapy for heart failure: with both treatments, cardiac output improves and the LV function curve shifts upward and to the left. For a given LV filling pressure, there is better cardiac output. (The patient moves from point A to point B.) With improved cardiac output spontaneous diuresis is possible with the patient moving to point C. This lowers pulmonary congestion while maintaining adequate cardiac output (point C).

common to use 100–150 µg/minute nitroglycerin. For initially hypertensive patients our target is a systolic blood pressure of 130–140 mmHg.

Catecholamines
Inotropic agents can be used in patients with pulmonary congestion and heart failure in addition to those with hypotension and shock (Table 6.6). A common indication for catecholamine treatment is low urine output. Low dose intravenous dopamine improves renal blood flow independent of cardiac effects, and may promote diuresis. Catecholamines and other inotropic agents improve cardiac output by increasing contractility (Fig. 6.6). As with afterload reduction, cardiac output is higher at any given level of LV filling pressure.

Theoretically, this approach has drawbacks. Improved overall function is achieved by making ischemic and recently injured muscle work harder. This would seemingly aggrevate ischemia, but careful study of treatment with inotropic agents during acute MI has uncovered no untoward effects. On the contrary, the catecholamine related increase in contractility produced a fall rather than an increase in coronary venous lactate, indicating less anaerobic metabolism. The explanation for this lies with the effect of inotropic therapy on overall cardiac efficiency. Improved contractility generates higher cardiac output, spontaneous diuresis, and a fall in LV volume (Fig. 6.6). This reduces myocardial oxygen demand via the LaPlace relationship:

wall tension = LV pressure × LV radius.

Myocardial oxygen demand is directly related to LV wall tension. As the radius (or volume) of the chamber declines with inotropic therapy, wall tension falls and so does oxygen demand (without necessarily changing developed LV pressure).

For these reasons, inotropic agents can be cautiously used to improve contractility and induce diuresis in patients with severe CHF during acute MI. There are a few considerations in choosing an inotropic agent. We would not use digoxin because of its long half-life and toxicity. Digoxin is used only to control ventricular rate in patients with MI who develop rapid atrial arrhythmias. At low doses, dopamine may improve renal blood flow. Dobutamine (Dobutrex®) is a pure inotropic agent with fewer noncardiac effects. It has less tendency than others to provoke ventricular arrhythmias. We avoid isoproterenol (Isuprel®), which may provoke ventricular ectopy, and levarterenol (Levophed®), which functions almost as a pure peripheral vasoconstrictor. These selective features of the catecholamines hold true only at low doses. Once the dose of any of the catecholamines is increased to high levels (above 10 μg/kg per minute), selective actions disappear and all work as pure vasoconstrictors.

A particularly effective combination is dopamine and dobutamine. Richard, et al., 1983 found that dopamine infusion rates above 10 μg/kg per minute caused an increase in LV filling pressure. When dopamine and dobutamine were combined, each at 7.5 μg/kg per minute, systolic blood pressure rose, but LV filling pressure decreased.

Patients with CHF and pulmonary congestion generally do not need high dose catecholamine therapy. More commonly, small doses are used to promote diuresis. Dopamine appears to be especially useful for its renal effects.

Cardiogenic shock

Before CCUs, the major cause of death with MI was VF. Early arrhythmia detection and DC cardioversion now make it rare for patients to die from isolated arrhythmias. Presently, the most common cause of death with MI is LV failure and cardiogenic shock. In the CITTS study we found that 6% of 253 patients treated with thrombolytic therapy within 4 hours of onset of pain died while in hospital; 12 of the 15 who died had cardiogenic shock or severe LV failure.

Before thrombolytic therapy, the incidence of cardiogenic shock among patients with acute MI was 10–12%. These patients had a 50% mortality rate within 10 hours of the onset of shock and an 80% mortality rate while in hospital. The clinical criteria for shock proposed by Killip (Killip class IV) include hypotension, oliguria, and mental obtundation (Table 2.2). Since shock can result from volume depletion as well as pump failure, it helps to get hemodynamic confirmation of LV failure by measuring pulmonary wedge pressure using a pulmonary artery floatation catheter. A commonly used hemodynamic definition of cardiogenic shock is systolic blood pressure less than 90 mmHg with a pulmonary wedge pressure >12 mmHg (although most with cardiogenic shock and heart failure have much higher wedge pressure). In one multicenter trial, 85% of patients meeting these hemodynamic criteria died. LV pump failure causing hypotension occurs most commonly in patients with anterior MI or those with a history of previous MI. Patients with shock usually have severe pulmonary congestion as well.

When evaluating a patient with shock or hypotension it is important to exclude conditions other than LV failure that can lower blood pressure (Table 6.7). Vasovagal reactions and hypotension are especially common, even in patients who are having acute MI. Those with inferior MI most commonly have increased vagal tone. Reperfusion leading to the Bezold–Jarish reflex with vagally mediated hypotension and bradycardia has been described above. Patients who have been ill for more than 1 day may have had reduced oral intake and have an element of volume depletion. This may be aggrevated by diuretic use in patients being treated for hypertension. The diagnosis of MI is usually obvious from symptoms and the ECG. But if the diagnosis is not clear, consider other causes of hypotension (Table 6.7).

RV infarction syndrome

The patient with hypotension and acute inferior MI and who has no pulmonary rales may have the RV infarction syndrome. Clinical findings have been reviewed in Chapter 3. Hemodynamic monitoring shows high right atrial pressure and low to normal pulmonary wedge pressure. The failing right ventricle is unable to

Table 6.7 A classification of hypotension in patients with suspected MI

Noncardiac causes of hypotension
Vasovagal reaction
Volume depletion
Septic shock
Hemorrhagic shock
Antiphylactic shock
Pheochromocytoma

Hypotension with chest pain, no MI
Pericardial tamponade
Tension pneumothorax
Pulmonary embolus
Aortic dissection

MI and shock
LV failure
LV rupture
Pericardial tamponade
RV infarction
Bezold—Jarish syndrome

push fluid through to the left side, and hypotension results from inadequate LV filling and low cardiac output. It is important to make the diagnosis of RV infarction quickly, as volume replacement may dramatically improve cardiac output. Treating such patients for "cardiogenic shock" with catecholamines is less effective, because the basic problem is inadequate filling of the left ventricle during diastole.

Treatment of shock

Prompt recognition of LV failure and shock is critical. The mortality risk within 10 hours may be as high as 50%. Your opportunity to help these patients could be limited to the first 6 hours after onset of shock. Later treatment is less effective. The following is an outline of critical steps in therapy of patients with hypotension and possible shock (Table 6.6).

Fluid replacement
A fluid challenge is a good initial maneuver for patients without dyspnea or pulmonary rales. It is directed at the patient with volume depletion, excessive vagal tone, or early RV infarction

syndrome. Give 200 ml normal saline quickly, intravenously, and repeat at 30 minute intervals. You must carefully monitor the chest examination during fluid loading. If the patient develops dyspnea, rales, or pulmonary congestion on the chest X-ray, stop the fluid infusion. Peripheral edema seen with RV infarction is not a contraindication to fluid loading. On the contrary, with RV infarction you must treat the right ventricle as a "passive conduit" and raise right-sided pressures enough to push fluid through to the left side. Patients often develop severe peripheral edema in the process. As RV function improves (or the RV "stiffens" with scar formation), usually within 2–3 weeks, peripheral edema may spontaneously resolve.

Thrombolytic therapy

The GISSI-1 trial comparing STK with placebo (Appendix 1) included 280 patients with cardiogenic shock; the mortality rate was 70% for patients treated with both placebo and intravenous STK. Thrombolytic therapy alone, therefore, may not be enough to save these patients. On the other hand, the Society for Cardiac Angiography Registry of patients treated with intracoronary STK found that patients with cardiogenic shock who had successful reperfusion had an 84% survival rate compared with 42% survival for those with a persistently occluded infarct artery. This finding is consistent with multiple small studies of reperfusion therapy (either pharmacologic or with angioplasty) showing that opening the infarct artery in patients with shock improves survival rates two to threefold.

Angiographic and pathologic studies of patients with cardiogenic shock show that patients with shock more commonly have total occlusion of the infarct artery and poor collateral flow to the infarct zone. For this reason rapid reperfusion may be especially important. Although not documented or specifically studied by random trials, a more rapidly acting thrombolytic agent like rt-PA may be especially useful in such patients.

The central Illinois experience is consistent with the literature; most patients with cardiogenic shock do not survive. Nevertheless, there are individual patients who improve dramatically with reperfusion, and early thrombolytic therapy offers them not only their best but perhaps their only chance.

Catecholamine therapy

Systemic hypotension must be treated and the goal is to raise systolic blood pressure to 70–90 mmHg. This hopefully will establish adequate perfusion of the myocardium, kidneys, and brain. Catecholamine therapy invariably is needed. As noted above, Richard, *et al.*, 1983 found that the combination of intravenous dobutamine 7.5 mg/kg per minute and dopamine 7.5 mg/kg per minute was better than high dose dopamine alone; the combination therapy raised cardiac output and blood pressure without raising LV filling pressure. Nonsurvivors usually declare themselves by their need for progressively higher doses of catecholamines to maintain blood pressure. Those requiring total doses above 20 μg/kg per minute and who have no urine output are almost certainly going to die.

Cardiac catheterization, angioplasty, and bypass surgery

A general discussion of timing of angiography and whether or not revascularization is needed, is the subject of Chapter 7. But let us consider the specific issues of revascularization in patients with cardiogenic shock. Studies of cardiogenic shock indicate that patients with open infarct arteries have improved survival. Thrombolytic therapy is a first step in this process. If prompt opening of the infarct artery is not apparent (indicated by an improvement in chest pain and the ECG and perhaps an increase in blood pressure), consider early angiography and angioplasty. Mortality rates are so high if the infarct artery remains closed that the patient has little to lose and much to gain.

Angioplasty may not help unless accomplished within 6 hours of the onset of shock. You have to decide quickly whether to take an aggressive, invasive approach. If you feel that the "heroic" effort is justified, start thrombolytic therapy and begin the move to the cardiac catheterization laboratory. Clinical judgment is required. A patient who obviously is dying should not undergo ambulance transfer. But if the patient is relatively stable on catecholamines, consider urgent transfer to the catheterization facility.

Do not expect magic with acute intervention. Death in the catheterization laboratory is not uncommon. In addition to shock, patients frequently have malignant ventricular arrhythmias. Many require intubation while in the catheterization laboratory.

Our first step is to put in the intra-aortic balloon pump (IABP) which improves cardiac output and reduces cardiac workload (Table 6.6). The IABP alone is not enough to save these patients; an early study of IABP support for cardiogenic shock found that it helped only those who also had an open infarct artery. As soon as the IABP is in place we proceed with angiography, then balloon dilatation if the artery has not opened. If the artery has opened and has fair antegrade flow, we might delay angioplasty. Abrupt reclosure of this unstable vessel could be fatal, and abrupt closure following angioplasty is much more frequent when it is performed early in the course of MI. The proper timing of angioplasty is based upon the appearance of the infarct artery. Clinical judgment based upon wide experience is critical. These are difficult cases, and are best avoided by inexperienced centers and operators.

Coronary artery bypass surgery was used in the early 1970s for patients with acute infarction and cardiogenic shock. More than 50% died during surgery and only 20% survived hospitalization. Opening the occluded artery is the critical initial step and must be done within 6 hours. Most centers will be able to accomplish this better in the catheterization laboratory than in the operating room. Patients with cardiogenic shock commonly have diffuse, multivessel, coronary disease. We have stabilized a number of such patients with early angioplasty, sending them for bypass surgery within the next 5 days. In a sense, this approach "selects survivors" for surgery. That makes sense to us, as good clinical judgment would favor keeping patients who are bound to die out of the operating room.

Selected reading

GISSI. Effectiveness of thrombolytic treatment in acute myocardial infarction. Lancet 1986;1:397–402.

ISAM Study Group. A prospective trial of intravenous streptokinase in acute myocardial infarction (ISAM): Mortality, morbidity and infarct size at 21 days. N Engl J Med 1986;324:1465–71.

ISIS-2 Collaborative Group. Randomized trial of intravenous streptokinase, oral aspirin, both, or neither among 17 183 cases of suspected acute myocardial infarction: ISIS-2*. J Am Coll Cardiol 1988;12: 3–13A.

Killip T, Kimball JT. Treatment of myocardial infarction in a coronary care unit. A two year experience with 250 patients. Am J Cardiol 1967;20:457–64.

Mathey DG, Kuck KH, Tilsner V, et al. Nonsurgical coronary artery recanalization in acute transmural myocardial infarction. Circulation 1981;63:489–97.

Mikell FL, Petrovich J, Snyder MC, et al. Reliability of Q-wave formation and QRS score in predicting regional and global left ventricular performance in acute myocardial infarction with successful reperfusion. Am J Cardiol 1986;57:923–26.

Richard C, Ricome JL, Rimailho A, et al. Combined hemodynamic effects of dopamine and dobutamine in cardiogenic shock. Circulation 1983;67:620–26.

Rogers WJ, Epstein AE, Arciniegas JG, *et al*. Special Report. Preliminary report: Effect of encainide and flecainide on mortality in a randomized trial of arrhythmia suppression after myocardial infarction. N Engl J Med 1989;321:406–12.

Taylor GJ, Bourland M, Mikell FL, *et al*. Dubious reliability of Q-wave formation in predicting new regional left ventricular akinesis after coronary artery bypass grafting. Am J Cardiol 1988;62:1299–1301.

Taylor GJ, Crampton RS, Gibson RS, *et al*. Prolonged QT interval at onset of acute myocardial infarction in predicting early phase ventricular tachycardia. Am Heart J 1981;102:16–24.

Taylor GJ, Mikell FL, Koester DL, *et al*. Comparison of intravenous tissue plasminogen activator (rt-PA) and streptokinase therapy for acute ST-segment elevation myocardial infarction: Improved regional wall motion in patients with anterior infarction treated with rt-PA. The Central Illinios Thrombolytic Therapy Study (CITTS) (Unpublished data).

Verstraete M, Bernard R, Bory M, *et al*. Randomized trial of i.v. recombinant tissue-type plasminogen activator versus i.v. streptokinase in acute myocardial infarction. Lancet 1985;1:842–47.

White HD, Norris RM, Brown MA, *et al*. Effect of intravenous streptokinase on left ventricular function and early survival after acute myocardial infarction. N Engl J Med 1987;317:850–55.

Wilcox RG, Von der Lippe G, Olsson CG, *et al*. Trial of tissue plasminogen activator for mortality reduction in acute myocardial infarction. Anglo-Scandinavian Study of Early Thrombolysis (ASSET). Lancet 1988;2:525–30.

Chapter 7

Interventional therapy after thrombolysis

Our approach to treating patients after thrombolytic therapy developed during the early 1980s. The treatment strategy was based on what we had been taught about unstable coronary syndromes and our clinical experience. The logic seemed clear. If you could identify a patient the day *before* his or her MI, angiography and revascularization obviously would be indicated. For a patient with a tight coronary artery stenosis, ragged plaque, and a 20% risk of arterial occlusion within the next month, revascularization would also be indicated and recommended, even if partial injury had occurred. Experience taught us to recommend revascularization for patients with non-Q wave infarction, a syndrome often associated with ragged, tight, and unstable coronary artery stenosis, with "incomplete" infarction, and with a high risk of subsequent occlusion and completion of MI.

The patient with recent thrombolytic therapy for acute MI appeared to be in a similar predicament. He or she demonstrated the instability of the coronary lesion by occluding the artery and had partial, not completed injury. Multiple trials showed reocclusion rates nearing 20%. We found it easy to recommend revascularization.

We have continued to gain confidence in and reaffirm our treatment strategy which includes early angiography and consideration of revascularization after thrombolytic therapy. It has not changed substantially since the early 1980s. Some current experts recommend medical therapy as the initial treatment approach after thrombolysis and believe that routine revascularization is unnecessary. We acknowledge that this is an area of controversy, but we point out that there are no long-term studies of patients who have received thrombolytic therapy and been managed medically. This chapter will review the controversy, and we freely admit that it presents our point of view.

We currently recommend that patients have cardiac catheterization within 1–2 days following thrombolytic therapy (Fig. 7.1).

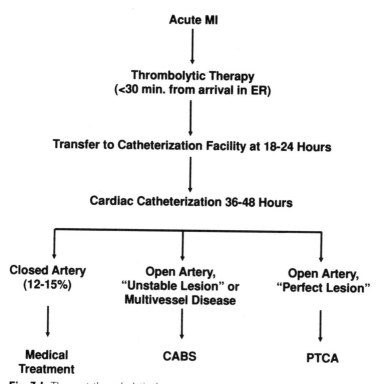

Fig. 7.1 The post-thrombolytic therapy treatment strategy currently followed at the Prairie Cardiovascular Center.

Until catheterization we treat them with aspirin and intravenous heparin. Frequently, other adjunctive therapies are used (Chapter 8). Patients who appear to have viable muscle in the infarct zone based upon clinical and angiographic findings, and who have a demonstrated critical stenosis of the infarct artery usually have a revascularization procedure. Using this approach, we have consistently offered revascularization to 60% of our patients; the proportion of patients treated with revascularization has not varied since 1982.

If you choose to use the treatment strategy described above, you can expect satisfactory short and long-term clinical results based upon our 10-year experience. We have reported the 6 year follow-up data for our initial series of 192 patients treated with thrombolytic therapy, early angiography, and early revascularization. Inhospital mortality was 6% (12 patients). During the next 6

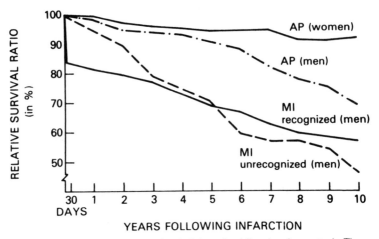

Fig. 7.2 The Framingham Study. Survival data after MI and angina pectoris. The survival ratio is relative to age-matched controls. (From Kannel WB, Sorlie P, McNamara PM. Am J Cardiol 1979;44:55.)

years, 21 of the 180 survivors (12%) died. Thus, cumulative 6-year mortality for these patients admitted with ST segment elevation infarction was 17% (33/192).

Without thrombolytic therapy, the 5-year mortality rate for patients having Q–wave MI was 45% (Kannel, *et al.*, 1979, Fig. 7.2). Our results with thrombolytic therapy and subsequent revascularization seem considerably better. When assessing efficacy of two different treatments, head-to-head comparative trials are desirable and we cannot cite the older studies ("historical controls") as proof that this strategy of thrombolysis and early revascularization is best. We are, however, satisfied with the validity of our experience. Using our approach, short and long-term survival results have been rewarding.

Not all of our patients have revascularization. In the CITTS study of 253 patients randomly treated with rt-PA or STK, 226 patients (88%) had an open infarct artery at catheterization the next day. A revascularization procedure was performed in 158 of them (62%); 94 had bypass surgery, and 64 had angioplasty. Table 7.1 outlines the reasons for using medical therapy rather than revascularization for the 95 patients who did not have bypass surgery or angioplasty. Apparent failure of thrombolytic therapy including a closed infarct artery and akinesis of the infarct zone, or an open infarct artery with suspected completed infarction was

Table 7.1 Indications for medical therapy in 95 of 253 patients after thrombolytic therapy (From CITTS trial)

Probable completed infarct	35
Closed infarct artery	14
Open infarct artery	21
Single vessel disease	14
Small infarct artery	
Minimal stenosis*	22
Died	11
Poor distal vessel	3
Poor general condition	2
Intracranial bleed	2
Patient refusal	6
	95

* Reduction of luminal diameter by <70%.

the most common reason for avoiding revascularization. Revascularization is best applied when there is salvage of myocardium, and it is best avoided in patients with completed infarction.

It is often difficult to ascertain infarct zone viability. Direct inspection of the heart during surgery indicates a spectrum of myocardial necrosis. Rather than "all or none," infarct zone injury is more often a case of "more or less." When the LV angiogram demonstrates that the infarct zone is still contracting, there is obviously live muscle in the area. Most patients after thrombolytic therapy have severe hypokinesis or akinesis of the infarct zone when the angiogram is performed within 4 days. A later study, done before hospital discharge, often shows some recovery of contractility in the infarct zone. The TPAT trial found that after thrombolytic therapy, infarct zone ejection fraction improved by 10 percentage points from day 1 to day 9 if the infarct artery was open.

Assessment of myocardial viability

There is no single clinical or angiographic feature which distinguishes nonviable from viable myocardium, and treatment decis-

Table 7.2 Assessment of myocardial viability after thrombolytic therapy

	Probably live muscle	Probably completed MI	Misleading findings
Clinical features	Early treatment	Late treatment	Equivocal pain response
	Good clinical response Pain relief Resolution of ST segment changes		
Laboratory findings	Early CK washout	Delayed elevation of CK	Equivocal ECG response
	Normal SA-ECG	Abnormal SA-ECG	Q waves
			Peak CK
Catheterization findings	Open infarct artery	Closed infarct artery	IZ hypokinesis or akinesis
	IZ contracts	Bulging IZ	
	Post-VPB contraction of IZ	Trabeculated IZ silhouette	
	Low LVEDP	Elevated LVEDP	

IZ, infarct zone.

ions are based upon multiple clinical variables (Table 7.2). Some assessment of myocardial viability is necessary in the first 2 days after infarction, as that is the time you must make decisions about subsequent treatment and particularly revascularization. It is a clinical decision that includes time to therapy and the patient's clinical response (Table 7.2). Positive clinical signs of reperfusion and salvage of myocardium include the abatement of chest pain and normalization of ST segments within 1–2 hours of thrombolytic therapy. An increase in ventricular ectopy and especially AIVR are common sentinels of reperfusion. The recurrence of chest pain or ST segment elevation subsequent to thrombolysis is an unfortunate but obvious indicator of residual, noninfarcted heart muscle. It is important to note that the presence of a Q wave does not prejudice us against recommending revascularization if there is other clinical evidence for myocardial salvage.

Cardiac catheterization findings are important in the assessment of myocardial viability. The ventriculogram obtained at cardiac catheterization is an especially helpful objective study in determining whether heart muscle salvage is sufficient enough to warrant recommendation for revascularization. As noted above (see p. 117), wall motion abnormalities are common. Bulging of the infarct segment both during diastole and systole may indicate completed infarction, and retention of normal LV shape suggests residual, viable muscle. Any inward motion of the infarct zone during systole suggests viable muscle. Improved infarct zone contraction with a post-VPB beat (the beat following the post-VPB pause) means viable muscle. We have noticed that increased trabeculation or haziness at the margin of the ventricular silhouette accompanies advanced injury. Absence of any motion of the epicardial coronary artery also indicates more severe injury. Patients with anterior MI who have LV-end-diastolic pressure (LVEDP) below 15–18 mmHg probably have viable muscle, and LVEDP above 25 mmHg is a bad sign.

The CK curve is especially useful. With reperfusion there is early CK washout. Instead of CK starting to rise at 12 hours and reaching its peak at 24 hours, thrombolysis causes a much earlier CK peak. Hohnloser and colleagues found that a CK peak ≤ 12 hours after thrombolytic therapy had a 98% positive predictive value in identifying patients with an open infarct artery 90 minutes after thrombolytic therapy. We routinely measure CK at 2, 4, 8, and 12 hours after thrombolytic therapy looking for early appearance of CK. While early CK appearance indicates reperfusion, reperfusion cannot be equated with absence of myocardial necrosis. Nevertheless, early reperfusion is an encouraging sign.

The signal averaged ECG (SA-ECG) may become a useful technique for assessing myocardial viability. This is a new test that is not widely available, but it is a simple, noninvasive technique. Low voltage "late potentials" occurring at the end of the QRS complex can be detected by epicardial surface electrograms (in the operating room), but cannot be identified by the surface ECG. These late potentials occur commonly in patients with complex ventricular arrhythmias, and may represent current in the protected focus responsible for re-entry (Chapter 6). The SA-ECG records these late potentials by adding a large number of QRS complexes using computer storage techniques and filtering environmental "noise" electronically. The composite QRS com-

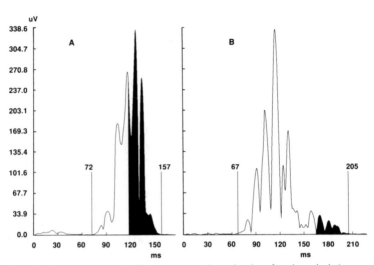

Fig. 7.3 Signal-averaged ECGs from two patients the day after thrombolytic therapy for acute anterior MI. Patient A is normal; voltage of the terminal 40 ms of the QRS complex is high. Patient B has "late potentials," low voltage current at the end of the QRS complex. The average voltage of the terminal 40 ms is low. These late potentials prolong the total duration of the QRS complex. Predischarge RNA showed LVEF 43% for patient A, 21% for patient B.

plex is huge, and the low voltage late potentials become visible. Thus, the SA-ECG allows us to detect the unusually low voltage late potentials using surface recording (Fig. 7.3).

Patients with late potentials on the SA-ECG are at higher risk for having complex ventricular arrhythmias. For example, the combination of a normal SA-ECG plus normal LV function effectively exclude VT in patients with syncope of uncertain cause. An abnormal SA-ECG after MI indicates a higher risk of complex ventricular arrhythmias.

Patients with an open infarct artery after thrombolytic therapy tend to have a normal SA-ECG. Those with a closed infarct artery more commonly have late potentials on the SA-ECG. The SA-ECG, like early washout of CK, may thus be a reliable test for early reperfusion. We have been even more interested in whether it can be used to assess myocardial salvage, and tested whether the SA-ECG would help us identify viable myocardium and select patients who should have revascualrization. We studied

Table 7.3 Signal averaged ECG and LVEF after thrombolytic therapy for acute MI

SA-ECG	LVEF (%)	
	Anterior MI	Inferior MI
Abnormal*	36 ± 8	54 ± 9
Normal	47 ± 14	57 ± 11
	$p < 0.01$	NS

* Terminal 40 ms r.m.s. voltage $<20 \mu V$.

100 patients having SA-ECG 1–2 days after MI and a RNA 8–10 days following MI. Patients with anterior MI and late potentials (an abnormal SA-ECG), had lower ejection fraction than patients with normal SA-ECG (Table 7.3). This pattern was not apparent in patients with inferior MI, possibly because baseline LVEF is normal in this group of patients.

An abnormal SA-ECG thus identifies patients with anterior infarction who have the largest infarction. It gives us this information 1–2 days after MI. We do not have to wait until day 8 to get the RNA. As an example of its usefulness, consider a patient with anterior MI who was treated 3½–4 hours after onset of pain, and who had an unclear clinical and ECG response to thrombolysis. He had an open infarct artery at catheterization but a large area of hypokinesis. A normal SA-ECG would suggest viable muscle in the anterior wall with some potential for recovery during the next 2 weeks; we would consider revascularization. An abnormal SA-ECG would leave us more pessimistic about chances for recovery of the anterior wall. In this case we probably would avoid early bypass surgery. We would wait a week, get a late RNA or echocardiogram, then make a decision about revascularization.

Transfer of patients

Our earliest trials with thrombolytic therapy required transfer of patients for *intracoronary* STK at the time of the acute infarction. When we switched to *intravenous* STK in 1983, patients were treated in the emergency department of the community hospital, and were then transferred directly from the emergency depart-

Table 7.4 Transport protocol following thrombolytic therapy for acute MI

Timing	The day after thrombolytic therapy
Transfer mode	Helicopter: complex ventricular ectopy, VT, hypotension, recurrent chest pain or reocclusion, pulmonary congestion, respiratory distress, otherwise unstable patient Ambulance: none of the above
Staffing	Two CCU nurses, possibly a respiratory therapist
Physician's role	Prior to departure with patient, the transport team calls the "receiving" cardiologist and gives report. At that time the cardiologist and transport team assume formal responsibility for patient management
Therapy during transport	Routine CCU orders plus intravenous heparin and lidocaine

ment to the referral center for urgent cardiac catheterization. We were fortunate during these earlier studies that no patient died during transfer. We did delay transfer for a small number of patients who were especially unstable, particularly those with excessive ventricular ectopy. Patients with large infarction were routinely transferred by helicopter. All patients were attended by CCU nurses during transfer. Time in transit generally was less than 1 hour.

Clinical experience teaches that patients are most unstable during the first 24 hours after thrombolytic therapy. Our current treatment protocol calls for transfer of patients the day after thrombolytic therapy (usually 18–24 hours after treatment), with cardiac catheterization planned 36–48 hours after treatment (Fig. 7.1). Transfer of patients 18–24 hours after therapy has been safe. Using this approach for more than 1000 patients we have had no deaths while in transit. Cardioversion in transit has been needed in <0.5% of these cases.

Our transfer protocol is outlined in Tables 7.4, 7.5. All patients are attended by CCU nurses. Almost all patients are on prophylactic, intravenous lidocaine. Those with largest infarction or who are clinically unstable are transferred by helicopter. By delaying transfer until the day after thrombolytic therapy, a smaller percentage of patients are felt to require helicopter transport. One reason patient transport has been statistically safe is our conscious effort to avoid transporting especially un-

Table 7.5 Transport orders

Obtain copies of patient records *including all ECGs* and *laboratory studies*

The receiving physician should be called and given a report

Intravenous line (preferably two) in place prior to transport. Have at least one extra i.v. site (heparin lock) for meds

Continuous cardiac monitor

Vital signs (heart rate, blood pressure, respirations) q 10–15 min

Oxygen per mask (as ordered) or nasal cannula @ 4 liters/min unless otherwise ordered

NTG 0.4 mg sublingual *prn* for chest pain if systolic blood pressure <90 mmHg. May repeat at 5 minute intervals as long as pain persists and systolic blood pressure >90 mmHg

Morphine Sulfate in 4 mg increments i.v. as needed for pain not relieved by 3 NTG tablets. Inject slowly and monitor blood pressure following each injection

Prophylactic lidocaine: 100 mg i.v. bolus, then 2 mg/min i.v. infusion

For patients who have received or are receiving peripheral i.v. thrombolytic therapy, follow the appropriate protocol

stable patients. The transport team routinely calls the receiving cardiologist before leaving with the patient. At that time the cardiologist and the transport team formally assume responsibility for patient management. The CCU nurses who are managing the patient during transport use standing orders that are similar to our CCU orders.

A subset that should be transferred *because of* cardiovascular instability includes patients with pump failure and cardiogenic shock. Acute revascularization may be their only chance. Emergency angioplasty is useful only if it can be performed within 6 hours of the onset of infarction. If you have a patient with cardiogenic shock who is otherwise healthy and appears to have a chance for survival, you must make a decision about "desperation" angiography and angioplasty early.

Cardiac catheterization

In the early 1970s cardiac catheterization was considered danger ous within 6 weeks of acute MI. At that time, angiographic studies done 8–12 days following infarction, just before hospital discharge, were considered bold and potentially dangerous. We have since learned that early angiography can be done safely. In our initial series of 1012 patients having thrombolytic therapy and early cardiac catheterization, we had no deaths in the catheterization laboratory with diagnostic angiography. This included 44 patients with severe LV failure and cardiogenic shock, many of whom subsequently died. But their deaths were not caused by the diagnostic angiogram. The only risk particularly related to early angiography was groin hematoma at the site of catheter insertion. This is a potentially significant problem and accounts for a majority of bleeding complications reported in most large series. In our study of 1012 patients, 4% had groin hematoma requiring intervention, and 0.7% needed transfusion. We are especially careful with arterial puncture technique and tend to use smaller diagnostic catheters (5 or 6 French).

Perhaps the greatest risk of early angiography is the temptation of the interventional cardiologist to do too much. The urge to dilate an infarct artery lesion that is marginally suitable for angioplasty may prove irresistible. Clinical judgment, experience, and restraint are exceedingly important qualities in this clinical setting.

Choice of revascularization procedures

Our choice of revascularization procedures was influenced by early experience with percutaneous transluminal coronary angioplasty (PTCA) in patients with recent thrombolytic therapy. Abrupt arterial closure after PTCA is more common in patients with recent thrombolytic therapy for MI than it is for patients having angioplasty for angina pectoris. A number of studies have found that coronary artery lesions that are markedly eccentric, have ragged surface or apparent plaque ulceration, or that have active thrombus, are at a higher risk for abrupt closure after angioplasty. By contrast, coronary artery stenoses that have smooth surfaces, a concentric "hour glass" configuration, and no apparent thrombus are low-risk lesions. They have better angiographic appearance after PTCA and less chance for abrupt closure. Catheterization within 48 hours of thrombolytic therapy for MI reveals a high proportion of coronary artery stenoses with the "high-risk" pattern.

In an effort to provide our patients with the most stable result possible we have reserved angioplasty for coronary arteries with "low-risk" lesions and have recommended coronary artery bypass surgery for those with high-risk lesions. Using this general approach, two-thirds of our patients having revascularization after thrombolytic therapy have bypass surgery and just one-third have PTCA.

This recommendation of bypass surgery as the initial revascularization technique for a majority of patients after thrombolytic therapy is substantially different from that promoted by the cardiology community in the last 5 years. For practical purposes, when cardiologists have discussed "revascularization" after thrombolytic therapy, they have meant "angioplasty." No formal trial incorporating revascularization, other than ours, has used bypass surgery as the predominant revascularization techniques. No trial has compared different revascularization techniques and none of the observational or randomized trials, apart from ours, has described late (5-year) follow-up.

The role of new catheter-based techniques including atherectomy, laser angioplasty, and intraluminal stenting is uncertain in patients after thrombolytic therapy. As atherectomy shaves off the ulcerated atheromatous plaque, it is an attractive possibility. In similar fashion, the results of laser angioplasty may be unaffected by the character of the plaque surface. Coronary artery stenting has also been suggested. However, the problem of thrombosis may be accentuated in the patient who has had recent MI and a greater tendency for thrombus formation in the unstable coronary artery. None of these techniques have been studied in patients having thrombolytic therapy.

Timing of revascularization

We have favored early rather than later revascularization; usually 2–3 days following acute MI. We are concerned about early reocclusion of the infarct artery and further injury. The sooner the artery is fixed, the better.

We delay PTCA for 36–48 hours, as angioplasty 48 hours after thrombolysis appears safer, with less abrupt closure, than angioplasty within 24 hours. Thrombus and possibly the thrombotic diathesis have had time to resolve. Futhermore, at 48 hours the stenosis that is viewed on the angiogram more likely represents atherosclerotic plaque and not thrombus.

Our surgical colleagues have observed that bypass surgery at 2–3 days, when the injured muscle is still relatively firm, may be

Table 7.6 Early bypass surgery after STK therapy for acute Q-Wave MI, 1981–83 (From Wellons, et al.)

	STK patients	Control* patients
Number	106	110
Time from MI to surgery	3 ± 2 days	—
Number of grafts	3.0 ± 1.4	3.6 ± 1.3
Units of blood	4 ± 3	4 ±2
Deaths	2.7%	2.7%
Days in hospital[†]	11 ± 5	10 ±4

* Consecutive series having surgery for standard indications.
[†] Total number of days in hospital including all preoperative days; 75% of control patients had angiography and surgery during the same admission.

better than operating at 10–14 days when necrosis is advanced and tissue is more friable. They also emphasize that from the vantage point of operative risk there is no need to wait. Waiting just prolongs hospitalization and recovery time. Surgery can be performed safely 2–3 days after thrombolytic therapy. Patients then experience a 1-week convalescence and are ready for discharge 10–12 days after acute MI. Using this approach for bypass surgery in patients treated with STK in 1981–83, we described a 2.7% mortality risk and average length of stay (from time of MI) of 11 ± 5 days (Table 7.6). More recently, in the CITTS trial, 98 of 253 patients had bypass surgery and just one died. That patient had cardiogenic shock prior to the operation.

Our experience with this treatment strategy of thrombolytic therapy, early angiography, and prompt revascularization may be the strongest argument in its favor. Our patients are doing well, and other studies have not influenced us to change our approach.

Clinical trials pertinent to revascularization after thrombolytic therapy

The problem of silent ischemia

Clinical trials that do not incorporate early revascularization often validate avoidance or delay of revascularization by a low reported incidence of "recurrent ischemia." A good example is the study by White, *et al.*, comparing STK and rt-PA with LV function as the major endpoint. Cardiac catheterization was performed 3 weeks after MI. They reported that fewer than 5% of their patients had "ischemic events" during the 3 weeks, suggesting that medical therapy (including heparin and aspirin) provided adequate protection for the other 95%.

We are beginning to understand that *symptomatic* ischemia may be the tip of the iceberg. During intracoronary STK therapy in the early 1980s, we commonly saw patients open the infarct artery in the catheterization laboratory, have improvement in ST segments and pain, then reocclude the artery with recurrence of ST segment elevation but without redeveloping chest pain.

More recently we have reported a series of patients having angioplasty after thrombolytic therapy who did not have chest pain during balloon occlusion of the infarct artery. As ischemia was induced by the balloon catheter, this study indicates the "potential" for silent ischemia after thrombolysis. There were 24 patients in this study who were treated with thrombolytic therapy less than 3 hours from the onset of chest pain, and who had an open infarct artery at the time of catheterization and angioplasty 2 days after MI. The angioplasty balloon was inflated in the coronary artery for 5 minutes producing total coronary artery occlusion (a relatively long balloon inflation time). During balloon inflation we monitored symptoms, pulmonary wedge pressure, and the ECG. All of the patients had new ST segment elevation during balloon inflation and a 3–10 mmHg rise in pulmonary wedge pressure (Fig. 7.4). ST segment elevation and a rise in plumonary wedge pressure indicate viable muscle in the infarct zone. Chest pain occurred in 5 of these 24 patients (21%) during balloon inflation. A comparison group of 20 patients without prior MI who had angioplasty had a similar rise in pulmonary wedge pressure and ST segments, and 70% of them developed angina during balloon occlusion of the coronary artery ($p < 0.003$). This study thus defines the potential for silent ischemia after successful thrombolysis; 79% of patients with apparently viable myocardium had infarct zone ischemia induced without having chest pain.

Further consider three interesting trials that have examined spontaneous or exercise-induced ischemia after thrombolytic therapy. Kayden, *et al.*, 1990 reported 33 patients who had ambulatory monitoring of LV function using a radionuclide technique, the nuclear stethoscope. Twelve of 33 patients had transi-

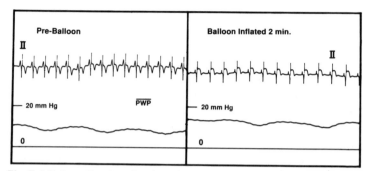

Fig. 7.4 Balloon dilatation after thrombolytic therapy. This 58-year-old man had thrombolytic therapy for acute inferior MI. After 2 minutes of balloon inflation monitor lead II showed ST segment elevation; pulmonary wedge pressure rose from 8 to 14 mmHg. Both of these findings indicate viable muscle in the infarct zone.

ent episodes of LV dysfunction with ejection fraction falling at least 5 percentage points for more than 1 minute. Only 2 of these 12 patients had associated chest pain and ECG changes. Follow-up 19 months later showed that cardiac events (unstable angina, MI, or death) occurred in 8 of the 12 patients with transient LV dysfunction (67%), compared with just 3 of 21 (14%) who did not have transient dysfunction. If the spontaneous and painless drop in ejection fraction represents silent ischemia, this study found it in 30% (10 of 33) of their patients.

Van der Wall and colleagues studied a group of 56 patients following thrombolytic therapy for acute MI who had a maximal exercise stress test just before hospital discharge. Ischemic ST segment depression was noted in 42 of the 56 patients (75%). Twenty of the 56 patients (36%), had no pain during a positive stress test indicating "silent ischemia."

Kwon and colleagues did continuous, 12-lead ECG monitoring in 31 patients who had thrombolytic therapy. Transient ST segment elevation occurred in 11 of their patients (32%). Eight patients had no symptoms with ST segment elevation suggesting spontaneous, silent ischemia in this subset of 26% (8 of 31).

These three clinical trials indicate that spontaneously occurring or exercise-induced silent ischemia occurs in 26–36% of patients who have had thrombolytic therapy. In each of these trials, "silent" ischemia was more common than symptomatic ischemia. Studies that report spontaneous recurrence of chest pain may thus underestimate the true recurrence rate of ischemia.

The TIMI-1 trial repeated cardiac catheterization just before hospital discharge and found occlusion of the previously open infarct artery in 21% of patients. About half of them had no symptoms indicating recurrent infarction.

Bleich, *et al.*, 1989 reported a study of 83 patients randomly allocated to heparin vs no heparin after rt-PA therapy. Angiography was performed in 2–3 days and showed infarct artery patency in 71% of patients on heparin, but in just 44% of those not anticoagulated. The authors assumed that initial patency rates were similar in the two study groups, but that reocclusion was more common in patients not anticoagulated. Interestingly, the rate of symptomatic ischemia or reinfarction was identical in the two groups. The authors conclude that heparin may ". . . decrease the incidence of clinically silent coronary reocclusion."

We used to believe that these patients with asymptomatic reocclusion of the infarct artery after thrombolytic therapy had no pain because the infarction was "complete," and there was no residual, viable muscle. We equated pain and muscle viability. With the new data indicating that silent ischemia is common, it is probable that many of these patients with reocclusion of the infarct artery had further ischemic injury, but did not feel it.

Some trials have relied on *late* coronary angiography or exercise testing to identify patients at risk for future ischemia. They may have missed silent ischemic injury, even in patients with an open artery at the time of follow-up catheterization. There probably are patients who have thrombolysis, subsequently have silent reocclusion with further injury, then reopen the artery. Late angiography would demonstrate the open artery, akinetic and probably dead myocardium, but with no clinical or angiographic hint of earlier events.

We consider the infarct artery unstable and dynamic in the days after thrombolysis, and we are concerned that spontaneous, silent ischemia may be common. Most available clinical trials have ignored this possibility.

Revascularization trials

TIMI-2

There have been few direct studies of early revascularization. The most influential of them is the TIMI-2 trial. In this study 3262 patients were treated with rt-PA within 4 hours of the onset of

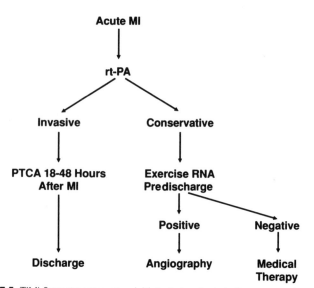

Fig. 7.5 TIMI-2 treatment protocol. Note that patients in the conservative wing had a predischarge exercise test which included a RNA. In order to justify treating your patients using the TIMI-2 conservative strategy, you must include a similar exercise study.

pain and were then randomly assigned to either "invasive" or "conservative" strategies (Fig. 7.5). The invasive group had angiography 18–48 hours after thrombolytic therapy with immediate PTCA if it appeared technically feasible. Conservatively-treated patients had cardiac catheterization and angioplasty only if ischemic pain recurred or if ischemia was provoked on a predischarge exercise test. The study found no difference in mortality or symptomatic reinfarction when comparing invasive and conservative groups. They also found no difference in LV function when measured by RNA at the time of hospital discharge.

When reported by the lay press, and as interpreted by most physicians, TIMI-2 was assumed to show that "revascularization and therefore, angiography, are unnecessary after thrombolytic therapy."

There are a number of problems with this interpretation of the TIMI-2 result. The first has to do with management of patients in the conservative wing of the study. These patients were not sent home after the heart attack without evaluation. All of them had an exercise RNA at the time of hospital discharge. Those with a positive exercise ECG and/or scan had angiography before discharge. *If you elect to follow the conservative treatment model of TIMI-2 you must incorporate a similar exercise study pre-discharge as a screen for potential ischemia.*

A simplistic interpretation of TIMI-2 tends to ignore the potential for future ischemia. The fact is that you cannot discharge these patients on medical therapy and expect a trouble-free clinical course. The TIMI-2A subgroup was the subject of a 1 year follow-up study. Revascularization was required by 39% of patients in the conservative wing, and the number of patients having angiography who did not require revascularization was not reported. Although treated conservative initially, patients in the conservative wing of TIMI-2 saw plenty of action during the next year.

Another problem with the TIMI-2 result is related to silent ischemia. As noted earlier, spontaneously occurring silent ischemia, and possibly silent ischemic injury may be common during the first week after thrombolytic therapy. Conservatively-treated patients may have had silent ischemic injury before the pre-discharge exercise study.

If this is the case, then why did the conservatively-treated patients do as well as those having "revascularization?" One explanation is that a large number of patients in the conservative wing "crossed over" and had revascularization. Another answer may be that TIMI-2 was not a trial of revascularization. Instead, it was a trial of culprit-lesion angioplasty. Revascularization was recommended for 1073 of 1636 patients (66%). Angioplasty was the initial technique used for 86% of patients who had revascularization; just 14% had bypass surgery. Arterial occlusion after angioplasty is more common in patients after thrombolytic therapy than it is for patients having angioplasty for angina pectoris. It is probable that some patients with unstable coronary artery lesions (marked eccentricity, ragged plaque, and plaque ulceration, or persistent thrombus) had temporary or permanent closure of dilated arteries following PTCA. At this stage after thrombolytic therapy for acute MI, a fair number of these occlusions would have been clinically silent.

What the TIMI-2 study does tell us is that early angioplasty after thrombolytic therapy is no better than medical treatment. It ignored the possibility that bypass surgery might protect myocardium after reperfusion. It did not compare surgical revascularization to angioplasty.

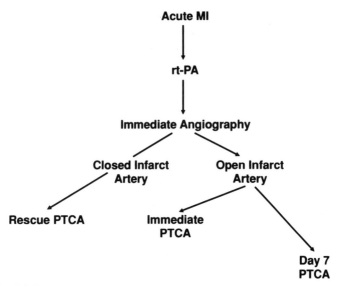

Fig. 7.6 TAMI phase I treatment protocol.

Our treatment strategy still includes revascularization in roughly 60% of our patients; two-thirds of these have bypass surgery and one-third have PTCA. We hope that by calling upon our experience in analyzing coronary angiograms we are able to "pick winners" for each of the revascularization techniques.

The TAMI-1 Trial

This study examined the role of emergency PTCA immediately after starting intravenous rt-PA for ST segment elevation infarction. Only patients who could be randomized within 4 hours of symptom onset were included. All patients in the trial had emergency angiography after receiving rt-PA (Fig. 7.6). All were treated with intravenous heparin, aspirin, and dipyridamole. Those with an open infarct artery who had a lesion suitable for PTCA were randomized to immediate PTCA or elective PTCA on day 7. Those with an occluded infarct artery at catheterization had immediate PTCA of the occluded artery ("salvage" or "rescue" angioplasty).

Patients who had an open infarct artery and immediate angioplasty had high success rate with PTCA (the artery looked better after PTCA). However, 9% of patients had abrupt closure of the artery during the procedure and could not be reopened;

7% were sent for emergency surgery, and 2% were managed medically. Patients allocated to the elective PTCA group 7–10 days later had a variable course. Only one-third had elective PTCA as planned. Twenty percent had recurrent chest pain, ECG changes, and required emergency revascularization (most in the first day), and 14% of the patients had improvement of the coronary stenosis and had a noncritical lesion at the time of catheterization 7–10 days later. When elective PTCA was performed a week after thrombolytic therapy there was less abrupt closure. Follow-up catheterization showed that reocclusion occurred in 11% of patients having immediate PTCA and 13% having elective PTCA.

Rescue angioplasty for the patients with a closed infarct artery at catheterization was initially successful in 85%, but there was a high complication rate. The hospital mortality rate was 10.5% (higher than other groups), and the rate of reclosure at follow-up catheterization was 29%. There was no significant improvement in global ejection fraction or regional wall motion at the time of follow-up catheterization in the group having rescue angioplasty. But the investigators noted that there were some individuals successes. The late survival rate for those who made it through hospitalization was good, consistent with other studies reporting that an open infarct artery increases long-term survival, even in the absence of measurable benefits on LV function.

Our treatment strategy differs substantially from that described in the TAMI study (Fig. 7.1). Rather than doing angiography immediately, we delay it for 24–48 hours. With this delay, the rate of abrupt closure with angioplasty is lower than when it is performed immediately. In a series of 64 patients in the CITTS trial who had angioplasty 2–3 days after thrombolytic therapy, abrupt closure resulted in angioplasty failure in just one (1.6%).

Our approach precludes the routine use of rescue angioplasty for patients who have not opened early with thrombolytic therapy. This is a small number of patients (12% of the CITTS series), not enough to justify emergency catheterization for all patients at the time of thrombolytic therapy. But patients with high-risk infarction should be considered for rescue PTCA, especially when there is heart failure or shock. When such patients fail to respond to thrombolytic therapy with relief of pain or improvement in the ECG, we recommend prompt referral for emergency catheterization and possible PTCA. If PTCA is to help patients with LV failure, it must be performed as early as possible, certainly within 6 hours of the onset of infarction. It is not worth doing 18–24 hours later. Thus, the decision for rescue angioplasty must be made early in the course of treatment, especially if patients require transfer to the catheterization laboratory facility.

Direct angioplasty for MI

Angioplasty is highly effective in patients with coronary occlusion and acute MI. It may work better than thrombolytic therapy, although there have been no trials comparing these two approaches. When a patient with MI arrives in our emergency room at a time when a catheterization laboratory is ready and available, we can open the infarct artery within 20–30 minutes of arrival in the catheterization laboratory with 90–95% certainty. This is not only faster but it produces a higher patency rate than can be achieved with thrombolytic agents. Direct angioplasty avoids the risk of bleeding complications associated with thrombolytic therapy.

The problem is that direct angioplasty is available for only a small minority of patients with MI. Hospitals without cardiac catheterization facilities would have to transfer patients with acute MI for angioplasty; they can better serve their patients with thrombolytic therapy. We have a sophisticated and efficient transport service, but gathering the CCU transfer team and ambulance or helicopter, reaching the patient, and then transporting him or her adds at least 2–3 hours before a catheterization laboratory procedure can be done. To do it any faster would require having the transport team and helicopter together, ready to take off 24 hours a day. We know of no hospital or referral system that is able to maintain this state of readiness.

Even when patients are admitted through our own emergency room, we frequently are unprepared for immediate catheterization and angioplasty. Late at night and on weekends, or when a catheterization laboratory is not readily available, it is faster to treat with thrombolytic agents in the emergency room.

Summary

Our current approach after thrombolytic therapy for acute MI is to transfer patients the day after therapy with angiography planned for the following day (36–48 hours after thrombolytic therapy). Patients with "perfect" or "low-risk" lesions that are suitable for angioplasty have PTCA or atherectomy. Those with ragged plaque or plaque ulceration, marked eccentricity or persistent thrombus, and patients with multivessel coronary disease, have coronary artery bypass surgery. Using this approach, 60% of our patients have a revascularization procedure (with two-thirds of these having bypass surgery).

As noted, this treatment strategy has worked well for us with good short and long-term survival rates and low morbidity and mortality rates with both PTCA and bypass surgery. By getting it all done within 2–3 days of MI, length of hospitalization is minimized, as is the total cost.

We are confident regarding this approach despite the TIMI-2 data. We do not feel that the TIMI-2 trial answers all questions about revascularization after thrombolytic therapy. Remember that if you elect to follow the TIMI-2 "conservative" model, you must include an exercise ECG/RNA before hospital discharge as a screen for high-risk patients. Failure to do this would constitute inadequate treatment according to TIMI-2. Furthermore, you must anticipate a "failure" of medical therapy and a need for revascularization in roughly 40% of your patients.

From a practical point of view, you need to work with the cardiology referral center in your area to develop a management strategy that you find comfortable. We recognize that this is an area of controversy. It is possible that future, randomized trials using revascularization strategies other than balloon angioplasty will offer further guidance.

Selected reading

Bleich SD, Nichols T, Schumacher R, *et al*. The role of heparin following coronary thrombolysis with tissue plasminogen activator (t-PA). Circulation 1989;80(Suppl II):II-113.

Califf RM, Topol EJ, George BS, *et al*. Characteristics and outcome of patients in whom reperfusion with intravenous tissue-type plasminogen activator fails: Results of the thrombolysis and angioplasty in myocardial infarction (TAMI) I trial. Circulation 1988;77:1090–99.

Chesebro JH, Knatterud G, Roberts R, *et al*. Thrombolysis in myocardial infarction (TIMI) trial, Phase I: a comparison between intravenous tissue plasminogen activator and intravenous streptokinase. Circulation 1987;76:142–54.

Hohnloser SH, Zabel M, Kasper W, Meinertz T, Just H. Assessment of coronary artery patency after thrombolytic therapy: Accurate prediction utilizing the combined analysis of three noninvasive markers. J Am Coll Cardiol 1991;18:44–9.

Kannel WB, Sorlie P, McNamara PM. Prognosis after initial myocardial infarction: The Framingham Study. Am J Cardiol 1979;44:53–9.

Kayden DS, Wackers, FJ, Zaret BL. Silent left ventricular dysfunction during routine activity after thrombolytic therapy for acute myocardial infarction. J Am Coll Cardiol 1990;15:1500–07.

Kwon K, Freedman B, Wilcox I, et al. The unstable ST segment early after thrombolysis for acute infarction and its usefulness as a marker of recurrent coronary occlusion. Am J Cardiol 1991;67:109–15.

Lange RA, Cigarroa RG, Wells PJ, Kremers MS, Hillis LD. Influence of anterograde flow in the infarct artery on the incidence of late potentials after acute myocardial infarction. Am J Cardiol 1990;65:554–8.

Morgan CD, Roberts RS, Haq A, et al. Coronary patency, infarct size and left ventricular function after thrombolytic therapy for acute myocardial infarction: Results from the tissue plasminogen activator: Toronto (TPAT) placebo-controlled trial. J Am Coll Cardiol 1991;17: 1451–57.

Ohman EM, Califf RM, Topol EJ, et al. Consequences of reocclusion after successful reperfusion therapy in acute myocardial infarction. Circulation 1990;82:781–91.

Rao A, Pratt C, Berke A, et al. TIMI trial-Phase I: Hemorrhagic manifestations and changes in plasma fibrinogen and the fibrinolytic system in patients treated with recombinant tissue plasminogen activator and streptokinase. J Am Coll Cardiol 1988;11:1–11.

Rogers WJ, Baim DS, Gore JM, et al. Comparison of immediate invasive, delayed invasive, and conservative strategies after tissue-type plasminogen activator. Results of the thrombolysis in myocardial infarction (TIMI) Phase II-A Trial*. Circulation 1990;81:1457–76.

Sheehan FH, Braunwald E, Canner P, et al. The effect of intravenous thrombolytic therapy on left ventricular function: a report on tissue-type plasminogen activator and streptokinase from the Thrombolysis in Myocardial Infarction (TIMI Phase I) Trial. Circulation 1987;75: 817–29.

Taylor GJ, Song A, Moses HW, et al. The primary care physician and thrombolytic therapy for acute myocardial infarction: Comparison of intravenous streptokinase in community hospitals and the tertiary referral center. J Am Board Fam Pract 1990;3:1–6.

Taylor GJ, Song A, Korsmeyer C, et al. Six year survival after thrombolysis for acute myocardial infarction. Circulation 1989;80(Suppl II): II–520.

Taylor GJ, Mikell FL, Koester DL, et al. Comparison of intravenous tissue plasminogen activator (rt-PA) and streptokinase therapy for acute ST-segment elevation myocardial infarction: Improved regional wall motion in patients with anterior infarction treated with rt-PA. CITTS (Unpublished data).

Taylor GJ, Mikell FL, Womack KA, et al. Nonfunctional nerves, live muscle: Silent ischemia after thrombolytic therapy for acute myocardial infarction (Unpublished data).

Taylor GJ, Mikell FL, Moses HW, et al. Intravenous versus intracoronary streptokinase therapy for acute myocardial infarction in community hospitals. Am J Cardiol 1984;54:256–60.

TIMI Study Group. Comparison of invasive and conservative strategies after treatment with intravenous tissue plasminogen activator in acute myocardial infarction. N Engl J Med 1989;320:618–27.

The TIMI Study Group. Special Report. The thrombolysis in myocardial infarction (TIMI) trial Phase I Findings. N Engl J Med 1985;312:932–36.

Topol EJ, Califf RM, George BS, Kereiakes DJ, Lee KL. The TAMI Study Group. Insights derived from the thrombolysis and angioplasty in myocardial infarction (TAMI) trials. J Am Coll Cardiol 1988;12:24–31A.

Van der Wall EE, Cats VM, Blokland AK, *et al.* The effects of diltiazem on cardiac function in silent ischemia after myocardial infarction. Am Heart J 1989;118:655–61.

Wellons HA, Schneider JA, Mikell FL, *et al.* Early operative intervention after thrombolytic therapy for acute myocardial infarction. J Vasc Surg 1985;2:186–91.

White HD, Rivers JT, Maslowski AH. Effect of intravenous streptokinase as compared with that of tissue plasminogen activator on left ventricular function after first myocardial infarction. N Engl J Med 1989;320:817–21.

Chapter 8
Adjunctive therapy

Thrombolytic therapy promotes myocardial salvage and survival during acute MI, but it has limitations. Not all patients have reperfusion. Myocardial injury develops rapidly during MI leaving many patients with substantial LV injury despite reperfusion. Reocclusion after thrombolytic therapy remains common. Adjunctive therapy, directed at these "shortcomings," may potentially improve the overall success rate of reperfusion therapy. This chapter will review drugs that have been proposed as adjuncts to thrombolytic therapy.

They include anticoagulants, aimed both at improving patency rates with thrombolysis, speeding the process of thrombolysis, and preserving arterial patency after reperfusion. Also included are agents that may directly promote myocardial salvage. This review does not include drugs used to treat complications of acute MI (Chapter 6).

We have limited data on adjunctive therapy as few of these agents have been studied in a setting of MI plus thrombolytic therapy (Table 8.1). It may be invalid to apply results from older studies of MI to patients who have had early reperfusion. We are careful to indicate where data are missing. At the same time, we make general recommendations about treatment based on what we do know.

Anticoagulant strategies

Heparin

Our current practice is to treat with full dose heparin (standing orders, Tables 5.2–5.4). The therapeutic goal is an activated partial thromboplastin time (aPTT) of 70–100 seconds measured 6–12 hours after starting heparin. If the aPTT is low, we give another 2000 U bolus of heparin and increase the hourly dose by 100–300 U/hour.

Table 8.1 Adjunctive therapy

	Facilitates thrombolysis	Reduces reinfarction (reocclusion)	Increases survival
Heparin	+	+	±
Aspirin	+	±	+
Beta blockers	0	+	±
Intravenous NTG Calcium blockers Magnesium ACE inhibitors	Not studied in patients with thrombolytic therapy for acute MI		

+ Yes.
± Uncertain, possible.
0 No.

Anticoagulation may aid the thrombolytic process in addition to preventing later rethrombosis and reocclusion. Deep arterial injury, including ruptured atherosclerotic plaque, exposes collagen and activates platelets leading to formation of thrombus. Fresh thrombus in turn promotes two processes: (1) further thrombosis as there is thrombin bound to the fresh clot, and (2) thrombolysis (Fig. 8.1). Thrombosis and thrombolysis are thus dynamic processes which occur simultaneously during the early stages of acute coronary artery occlusion. Blocking active and ongoing thrombosis with antithrombin agents such as heparin would tilt the balance in favor of thrombolysis (Fig. 8.1).

Also recall that each of the currently approved thrombolytic agents has been shown to activate platelets and other clotting mechanisms; an apparent rebound, prothrombotic effect. This effect may be blocked by anticoagulants given early in the course of thrombolytic therapy.

There have been clinical trials of heparin after thrombolytic therapy which have examined both arterial patency and clinical outcomes (including reinfarction and death). Heparin dosing and route of administration have been controversial. It is possible that comparative trials of STK and rt-PA have been influenced by the heparin dosing schedules. The clinical trials summarized in Figure 8.2 are commonly cited by proponents of full dose, intravenous heparin after thrombolytic therapy. All of these studies were done

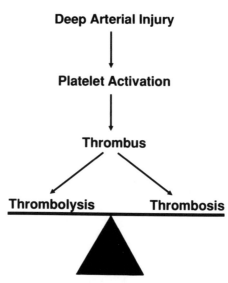

Deep Arterial Injury

↓

Platelet Activation

↓

Thrombus

Thrombolysis   **Thrombosis**

Fig. 8.1 Deep arterial injury exposes collagen resulting in platelet activation. Thrombus is formed and this simultaneously initiates further thrombosis and the process of thrombolysis. There is a dynamic equilibrium between thrombolysis and thrombosis. If one is inhibited, the other may predominate.

with rt-PA, used intravenous heparin, and examined arterial patency.

The TAMI-3 trial compared heparin with no heparin. Coronary angiography was performed 90 minutes after rt-PA treatment. Heparin had no beneficial effect on infarct artery patency. The conclusion was that early, 90 minute patency depends upon the efficacy of the thrombolytic agent and is not influenced by heparin. Three other studies examined the effect of heparin on patency when catheterization was performed between 18 hours and 4 days after thrombolytic therapy (Fig. 8.2). Each of these trials started intravenous heparin with thrombolytic therapy; the dose was adjusted so that aPTT was 1.5–2 × normal. Each of these three trials showed significantly higher patency in groups treated with heparin.

The Australian Heart Foundation trial was different. All patients in this study received intravenous heparin for 24 hours. After that, patients were randomly assigned to treatment with either intravenous heparin therapy or a combination of aspirin and dipyridamole. There was no difference in late infarct artery patency between the heparin and antiplatelet therapy groups.

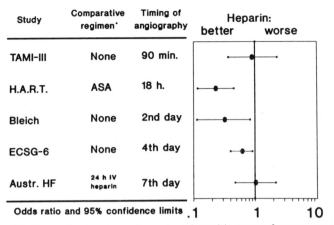

Fig. 8.2 Five randomized trials of heparin and arterial patency after treatment with rt-PA. (From Prins MH, Hirsh J. Am J Cardiol 1991;67:7A.)

Proponents of rt-PA have reviewed these studies which indicate an important interaction between heparin and rt-PA therapy and conclude that heparin is necessary to maintain infarct artery patency from 18 hours to 4 days after rt-PA therapy. While STK and APSAC have not been studied in similar trials, these agents deplete circulating fibrinogen producing a hypocoagulable state that is assumed to protect patients during the 24 hours after thrombolytic therapy. Since rt-PA has less effect on fibrinogen, *early* rethrombosis of the infarct artery is more likely with this agent.

Later rethrombosis may also be less common with fibrinogen-depleting agents (STK and APSAC). A hypocoagulable state for 24–36 hours after reperfusion may allow more complete resolution of thrombus, less accumulation of fresh thrombus and, therefore, a more stable plaque surface for a period of days.

Studies comparing rt-PA and STK which have not protected patients with full dose heparin may have missed an added benefit of rt-PA because of the higher rate of early or later reocclusion with this agent. The absence of heparin therapy is the major criticism of these trials (GISSI-2 and ISIS-3). The ongoing GUSTO trial uses full dose, intravenous heparin for all patients receiving rt-PA. One wing of this study will compare subcutaneous and intravenous heparin in patients treated with STK.

Table 8.2 Influence of subcutaneous heparin on mortality

| | Mortality | | |
Drug/study	Heparin	No heparin	p value
STK			
SCATI	10/218 (4.5%)	19/215 (8.8%)	p = 0.05
GISSI-2	254/5037 (5%)	311/5037 (6.2%)	p = 0.015
rt-PA			
GISSI-2	294/4988 (5.9%)	298/5047 (5.9%)	NS

Multiple studies (GISSI-2, SCATI, TAMI-3, Bleich, ECSG-6; note Appendix 1) have examined the effect of intravenous heparin on recurrence of ischemic symptoms or clinical reinfarction. None of them found any difference. It is hard to interpret this, as none of these studies addressed the issue of silent ischemia and silent ischemic injury which may be common after thrombolytic therapy (for a discussion of the silent ischemic issue, see Chapter 7).

Survival with and without *subcutaneous* heparin therapy was studied by GISSI-2 and SCATI (Table 8.2). Interestingly, heparin appeared to favorably influence mortality in patients treated with STK in both SCATI and GISSI-2, even though heparin was given subcutaneously in these studies. On the other hand, survival with rt-PA therapy was no different in patients treated with subcutaneous heparin (GISSI-2). It is possible that an antithrombin therapy more potent than subcutaneous heparin is needed to protect any gains achieved with rt-PA.

Bleeding complications increase when heparin is added. In the GISSI-2 trial, the risk of minor and severe bleeding doubled with subcutaneous heparin therapy. A similar trend was seen in the ISIS-3 trial with subcutaneous heparin. About 10% of patients treated in the ISIS-3 trial were given intravenous heparin, not by study design, but by physician preference; most of these patients were treated in the United States. The risk of intracranial bleeding was higher in the patients treated with intravenous heparin. The ISIS-3 investigators commented that the higher intracranial bleeding risk may off-set any small reduction in cardiac mortality achieved with intravenous rather than subcutaneous heparin. This issue may be settled by the GUSTO trial.

The route of heparin administration thus remains controversial at this time. Both experimental and clinical studies have shown that aPTT >50 seconds reduces the recurrence of myocardial ischemia in patients who have had thrombolytic therapy, just as it reduces the recurrence rate of thromboemboli in patients with venous disease. It is difficult to achieve this therapeutic level with subcutaneous heparin. One study treated patients with 15 000 U *subcutaneous* heparin twice a day after an initial intravenous bolus of 5000 U, and less than half the patients had a therapeutic aPTT during the first 24 hours. By contrast, most patients given 5000 U heparin intravenously followed by continuous infusion of approximately 30 000 U over 24 hours have a therapeutic effect during the first day.

In addition to preventing recurrent thrombosis and reocclusion of infarct arteries, heparin is also beneficial in preventing LV mural thrombus. The SCATI trial specifically addressed this point with predischarge echocardiograms on all patients with first anterior MI. Mural thrombus was observed in 18% of those who were treated with subcutaneous heparin and in 37% of patients who were not treated.

Other antithrombin drugs

Thrombus formation after deep arterial injury (including atheromatous plaque rupture) involves a complex interaction of collagen, platelets, and thrombin (Fig. 8.3). Platelets are activated following contact with collagen. Both activated platelets and collagen promote conversion of prothrombin to thrombin. Thrombin, in turn, converts fibrinogen to fibrin. But it appears that the thrombin that is bound to the developing thrombus, also *activates platelets*, and this action of clot-bound thrombin may be as important as its effect on fibrinogen in promoting ongoing thrombosis after deep arterial injury. Platelet activation by thrombin has been inferred from studies of hirudin and argatroban, antithrombin agents which have no direct antiplatelet activity *in vitro*. But use of these agents *in vivo* has been found to limit platelet deposition. In fact, the antithrombin drugs were more effective than specific platelet inhibitors in reducing platelet activation and deposition in injured arteries. Thus, there appears to be a role for thrombin in activation of platelets and production of arterial thrombus after deep arterial injury.

Heparin is the time-tested antithrombotic drug, but it does

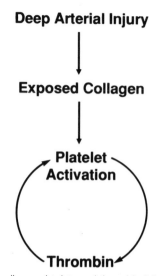

Deep Arterial Injury

Exposed Collagen

Platelet Activation

Thrombin

Fig. 8.3 Interaction of collagen, platelets, and thrombin following deep arterial injury. Exposed collagen activates coagulation factors producing thrombin. It also activates platelets causing aggregation, then release of ADP, thromboxane, and serotonin. These substances further stimulate clotting factors producing more thrombin. Not widely appreciated is the profound effect of thrombin on platelet function. Studies of specific and powerful thrombin inhibitors, which have no intrinsic antiplatelet activity, found that these drugs have a greater effect on platelet aggregation *in vivo* than specific antiplatelet drugs. In a setting of deep arterial injury thrombin may be the most powerful activator of platelets.

not completely inhibit thrombin even at unusually high doses (>500 mg/kg over 1 hour). This is the reason for interest in new, specific, and more potent thrombin inhibitors such as hirudin and argatroban. More effective antithrombin activity is hoped to block more completely thrombin-mediated platelet activation. In experimental preparations, these agents have been found to be much more effective in preventing thrombosis following deep arterial injury (including placement of metallic intra-arterial stents) than either aspirin or heparin.

Heparin is less effective than the newer drugs. One reason is the large size of the heparin molecule. Fresh or residual thrombus contains active thrombin which is fibrin-bound, and the large heparin–antithrombin III complex cannot reach it. In addition, arterial thrombus contains substances which inhibit heparin.

In contrast, hirudin is a much smaller molecule than heparin and has no natural inhibitors. It thus works more effectively on fibrin-bound thrombin. This may be especially important, as the residual thrombus which contains thrombin and which adheres to the ruptured plaque after thrombolytic therapy may be more thrombogenic than deep arterial injury (exposed collagen) alone. Experimental studies indicate that this is especially true when there is tight stenosis of the vessel.

Antiplatelet therapy/aspirin

Our current approach follows the ISIS-2 recommendation. Our standing orders call for immediate therapy with 160 mg chewed aspirin (2 baby aspirin, Tables 5.2–5.4) regardless of which thrombolytic agent is used. Patients are then treated with one adult aspirin (325 mg) daily.

Platelet activation is the earliest step in thrombus formation. Platelets adhere to exposed collagen and release contents of their granules including thromboxane A_2, serotonin, and ADP. These substances promote further platelet aggregation and release, amplifying the platelet effect. Animal studies have shown that the rate of thrombolysis is faster when platelet activation is blocked by specific inhibitors of thromboxane A_2 and serotonin receptors. In these studies, animals treated with rt-PA and heparin alone had a pattern of cyclical reperfusion, then reocclusion early after administration of rt-PA and heparin. Reocclusion appeared due to transient platelet plug formation. This cyclical flow variation was prevented by platelet inactivation with thromboxane and serotonin receptor antagonists. Time to lysis of the thrombus was accelerated by the antiplatelet drugs, probably by preventing ongoing platelet activation during the early stages of thrombolysis (Fig. 8.1).

This is an important way to think about antiplatelet agents as well as antithrombin therapy. Anticoagulation obviously is important in preventing reocclusion following thrombolysis, but anticoagulants also work during thrombolysis to accelerate the thrombolytic process. This may explain the somewhat surprising effect of aspirin on survival in the ISIS-2 trial (Fig. 8.4). In this large and important study, patients chewed 160 mg aspirin immediately after identification of MI. Aspirin alone provided a survival effect similar to that seen with STK alone. There was a strong, synergistic effect of the two drugs together. What aspirin probably did was block ongoing thrombosis leaving drug induced or naturally occurring thrombolysis unopposed (Fig. 8.1).

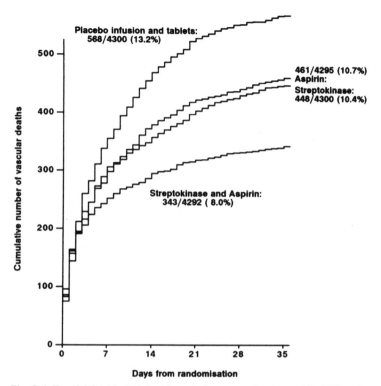

Fig. 8.4 The ISIS-2 trial which had four study groups: placebo, aspirin, STK, and STK + aspirin. This figure is perhaps the most widely reproduced in the literature on thrombolytic therapy. The results secure the role of aspirin/antiplatelet therapy as an important adjunct to thrombolysis. (From ISIS-2 Collaborative Group. Randomised trial of intravenous streptokinase, oral aspirin, both, or neither among 17 187 cases of suspected acute myocardial infarction: ISIS-2. Lancet 1988;2:349–60.)

The only study to address aspirin therapy in combination with rt-PA was HART (Appendix 1). In this study patients treated with rt-PA plus heparin had a 90-minute arterial patency rate of 82% compared with 52% in patients treated with rt-PA plus aspirin. Follow-up angiography 1 week later showed a patency rate of 90% in both groups. The study did not evaluate rt-PA alone, or rt-PA plus heparin and aspirin.

A number of experimental antiplatelet agents are being investigated as possible adjuncts. These include thromboxane synthesis inhibitors, thromboxane receptor antagonists, serotonin receptor antagonists, and monoclonal antibodies to platelet glycoprotein

Table 8.3 Intravenous and oral beta adrenergic blockers during acute MI

Patient selection	Acute MI, <12 hrs from onset of pain
Exclusion criteria	Heart failure, systolic blood pressure <100 mmHg, heart rate <60/min, bradyarrhythmia or heart block, asthma or obstructive lung disease
Drug regimen	Metoprolol 5 mg i.v. at 5 min intervals ×3 doses Then 100 mg p.o. q.i.d. for 48 hours Then 100 mg p.o. b.i.d. Atenolol 5 mg i.v. over 5 min Repeat i.v. Atenolol 5 mg dose 10 min later Atenolol 50 mg p.o. 10 min later Then 50–100 mg daily
Duration of treatment	Intravenous therapy initially, oral therapy long term
Potential benefits	Blunts catecholamine effect reducing heart rate, blood pressure, and contractility. This reduces infarct size. Improved survival has been related to lower incidence of VF and LV rupture

IIb/IIIa receptors. No clinical data are available, but studies in animal models are encouraging.

Beta adrenergic blockers

Patients with acute MI often respond to intravenous beta blockade with a dramatic improvement in chest pain and resolution of ST segment elevation. Our current practice is to use intravenous metoprolol or atenolol during acute MI whenever possible and regardless of whether or not thrombolytic therapy is given (Table 8.3). We have not included beta blockade in our standing orders for thrombolytic therapy (Chapter 5). Like thrombolytic therapy, intravenous beta blockade is most effective when applied early in the course of MI.

Patients with acute MI have high circulating catecholamine levels. The resulting increase in heart rate, blood pressure, and contractility all raise myocardial oxygen demand. Beta blockers reduce myocardial oxygen demand by blunting all of these actions of catecholamines. By reducing wall stress, beta blockers may also help prevent myocardial rupture. VF is less common in patients with MI treated with intravenous beta blockers, and survival

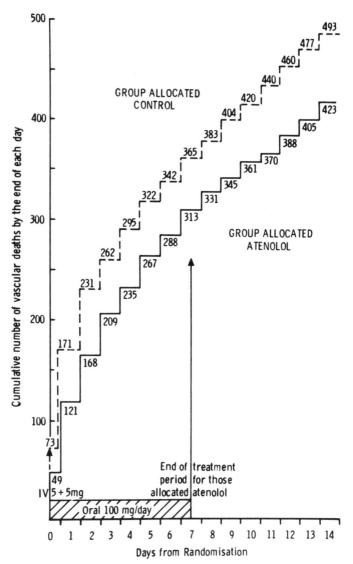

Fig. 8.5 The ISIS-1 study of atenolol following acute MI. This was *not* a study of thrombolytic therapy. There is a significant reduction in mortality noted within the first two days of acute MI. Survival curves were parallel after that point. (From ISIS-1 Collaborative Group. Randomised trial of intravenous atenolol among 16 027 cases of suspected acute myocardial infarction: ISIS-1. Lancet 1986;2: 57–66.)

benefits documented by large trials can be attributed to the lower incidence of VF and myocardial rupture.

Data are now available from 28 randomized trials of acute MI in the prethrombolytic therapy era including over 27 000 patients. Average reduction in mortality with beta blocker therapy is 13–15%, with greatest benefit seen during the first 2 days after MI (Fig. 8.5). By contrast, GISSI-1 and ISIS-2 found that thrombolytic therapy did not improve survival within the first 24 hours. This suggests a complementary role for intravenous beta blocker and thrombolytic therapy.

There has been just one small study of beta blocker therapy in patients who were also treated with thrombolytic therapy, TIMI-2. It did not demonstrate any survival benefit with intravenous metoprolol. However, there was a significant reduction in early, nonfatal reinfarction (16/696 vs 31/694, $p < 0.05$), and a similar reduction in symptomatic ischemic episodes. The study did not address the issue of silent ischemia.

Studies of long-term beta blocker therapy in patients with acute MI treated after hospital discharge have shown that late mortality is reduced by roughly 25%. These large trials from the 1970s did not include angiography, thrombolytic therapy, or revascularization. A precise knowledge of coronary artery anatomy allows us to identify patients at high risk for recurrent ischemia, and such patients would benefit from beta blocker therapy. If early revascularization negates the possibility of recurrent ischemia, there would be less need for long-term beta blocker therapy. There are no studies indicating that patients who have had bypass surgery or angioplasty are helped by beta blocker therapy.

An argument can be made to include beta blockers in the therapeutic regimen for patients treated "conservatively" after thrombolytic therapy (without revascularization).

Nitroglycerin

Jugdutt, et al. (1988, 1989) have shown that intravenous nitroglycerin reduces the size of MI and also prevents infarct expansion (Tables 8.1, 8.4). These effects reduce morbidity and possibly mortality. Mechanisms of action include venodilatation, reduced venous return to the heart, lower "preload," and reduced force of contraction. This limits myocardial oxygen demand, thereby reducing infarct size. Myocardial oxygen supply may be raised by dilatation of coronary artery collaterals.

Table 8.4 Intravenous nitroglycerin during acute MI

Patient selection	Acute MI, <12 hours from onset of pain, mean arterial pressure >80 mmHg (systolic blood pressure >105–110 mmHg)
Exclusion criteria	Cardiogenic shock, mean arterial pressure <80 mmHg
Dose	Start with 5 µg/min i.v. Increase the dose to lower mean arterial pressure by 10% in normotensive patients, 30% in hypertensive patients Do not lower *mean* pressure below 80 mmHg (or systolic pressure below 105–110 mmHg)
Duration	Treat with i.v. nitroglycerin for 48 hours
Potential benefits	Low dose nitroglycerin reduces preload, possibly afterload and may improve flow through coronary collaterals. The result is less infarct expansion and LV dilatation, and improved LV function

A critical feature of these studies was the titration of intravenous nitroglycerin to specific hemodynamic endpoints aimed at reducing preload, *but without lowering mean arterial pressure below 80 mmHg (systolic blood pressure 105–110 mmHg)*. When blood pressure was lowered further, the beneficial effect was not observed, possibly because of reduced coronary artery perfusion pressure. In these studies, the average dose of intravenous nitroglycerin was 45 µg/minute (range 4–192 µg/minute). Greatest myocardial salvage was achieved when therapy was begun within 4 hours of onset of pain. Hypotension was infrequent with this cautious dosing regimen. Therapy was adequately monitored by nurses using standard blood pressure monitoring equipment. Patients with inferior MI were more sensitive to blood pressure lowering effects of intravenous nitroglycerin and needed more careful monitoring.

In addition to potential salutary effects of nitrates on LV function and myocardial oxygen demand, nitrates may help prevent reocclusion after thrombolysis. The infarct artery usually has tight stenosis, and coronary vasospasm may contribute to reocclusion. But all of this is speculation. Intravenous nitroglycerin has not been studied in patients with acute MI and thrombolytic therapy. It is highly effective in treatment of unstable angina pectoris, and clinicians commonly approach the post-thrombolytic therapy patient in similar fashion. A fair percentage of patients transferred to our service from community hospitals after thrombolytic therapy are on intravenous nitroglycerin, and we continue it. We find it especially useful in patients with large MI and with elevated blood pressure (Table 8.4).

Calcium channel blockers

A number of random trials have studied calcium channel blockers in patients following MI and have found no beneficial effect on mortality, infarct size, or LV function. For the secondary prevention of MI after an initial infarction, beta blocker therapy and aspirin appear more effective.

Two studies have examined the effect of diltiazem (Cardizem®) on patients with non-Q wave MI. The Diltiazem Reinfarction Study randomly treated patients with diltiazem (90 mg every 6 hours) or placebo, and observed them for 14 days. The rate of reinfarction during the 2 weeks was 51% less for the diltiazem group. The incidence of angina was also reduced by diltiazem.

The Multicenter Diltiazem Postinfarction Trial followed patients for an average of 2 years and observed a reduction in cardiac events (death or recurrent MI) with diltiazem 240 mg/day. The beneficial effect was limited to patients with good LV function. (Patients with heart failure or LVEF <40% had *more* cardiac events with diltiazem.) This benefit was maintained at 4 years.

Patients with non-Q wave infarction have much in common with patients who have had recent thrombolytic therapy for ST segment elevation MI. At angiography both groups have tight and ragged coronary artery lesions, and both have "incomplete" or partial injury. There has been no study of adequate size to detect a potential benefit of calcium antagonist therapy after reperfusion. We feel that the issue is as yet unstudied. Our clinical impression is that patients after thrombolytic therapy have "irritable" arteries that are prone to developing spasm. Theoretically, calcium channel blockers should help. They may be especially helpful for patients who are treated medically who do not have early angiography or revascularization.

Another potential benefit of calcium antagonists during reperfusion therapy is a direct effect of the drugs on mechanisms of cell death. A rise in intracellular calcium has been demonstrated in experimental animals with coronary artery occlusion, then reperfusion. These studies have demonstrated a number of deleterious effects of increased intracellular calcium levels including depletion of high energy phosphate stores, activation of cytotoxic enzymes, changing functional capabilities of cellular proteins, and development of "late potentials" on the signal averaged ECG. High levels of intracellular calcium may be responsible for "contraction-band necrosis," the specific pathologic pattern seen with reperfusion. Preliminary studies have indicated a role for calcium antagonists as myocardial protectors during ischemic arrest and cardiopulmonary bypass. More work examining a possible role for calcium antagonists during acute MI and reperfusion is needed.

In a review of all randomized trials using calcium antagonists for acute MI, Yusuf, *et al.* (1991) noted a trend toward higher mortality among patients treated with nifedipine. By contrast, trials using diltiazem and verapamil showed a trend toward fewer reinfarctions. The major difference between nifedipine and the other agents is that nifedipine causes a reflex increase in heart rate and the others decrease heart rate. There is a suggestion that drugs which reduce heart rate, including beta blockers, may have more salutary effects on patients after MI. Because of these data, we would suggest concomitant use of beta blocker therapy with nifedipine when it is being used to control or prevent angina pectoris following acute MI.

Magnesium

Magnesium has been neglected. Most hospitals do not measure it as part of the routine admission panel. There are good data relating hypomagnesemia to cardiac arrhythmias in patients with myocardial ischemia or recent heart surgery. Reduced magnesium levels are common in patients on diuretic therapy. Thiazide diuretics, which lower serum potassium, have a similar effect on magnesium, depleting serum and intracellular stores.

Patients with acute MI often have transient low magnesium levels. This may contribute to prolongation of the QT interval that often occurs with early infarction. Prolonged QT interval after MI has an association with increased ventricular ectopy (Chapter 6).

There have been three random trials of magnesium infusion during acute MI (without thrombolytic therapy). In each, there was a 50% reduction in the incidence of ventricular arrhythmias. One of the trials showed improved survival. These data indicate,

Table 8.5 Intravenous magnesium during acute MI

Indications	Serum magnesium <1.8 mg/dl, torsade de pointes, frequent PVCs plus borderline low magnesium
Cautions	Hypotension, heart block, renal failure
Dose	Magnesium sulfate 1 g i.v. q 1 h ×4 doses Then magnesium gluconate 500 mg p.o. t.i.d. Repeat serum magnesium daily ×2
Comment	Goal: serum magnesium 2.0–2.5 mg/dl Depressed serum magnesium is commonly found in clinical settings that cause hypokalemia (especially diuretic therapy)

PVC, premature ventricular contraction.

at the least, that magnesium should be replaced if it is low. In our practice, we treat patients with magnesium ≤1.8 mg/dl with intravenous magnesium sulfate (Table 8.5). The goal is a magnesium level of 2.0–2.5 mg/dl.

Apart from its effect on cardiac arrhythmias, magnesium may prevent vascular spasm, favorably influence collateral flow, and inhibit platelet aggregation. It has not been specifically studied as an adjunct to thrombolytic therapy for acute MI, but is being included as a wing of the ISIS-4 trial.

Angiotensin converting enzyme (ACE) inhibitors

Angiotensin is present in the epicardial coronary arteries as well as the small, resistance vessels downstream. Conversion of angiotensin I to angiotensin II is possible at both locations. Angiotensin II is a potent vasoconstrictor and may reduce myocardial oxygen supply (coronary blood flow) at the time of acute infarction. Blocking production of angiotensin II in experimental animals has been shown to limit infarct size. There have been no clinical trials of ACE inhibitors in acute MI or as an adjunct to thrombolytic therapy.

Afterload reduction with captopril has been shown to reduce infarct expansion in patients who have had large MI with LVEF <40–45% (Pfeffer, *et al.*, 1988, Sharpe, *et al.*, 1988). In these randomized, placebo-controlled studies, patients had repeat echocardiograms during the year after MI. Those receiving captopril had less infarct expansion and LV dilatation. It should

Table 8.6 ACE inhibitors following MI

Patient selection	Patients with acute MI with substantial LV injury (LVEF <45%)
Exclusion criteria	Systolic blood pressure <105–110 mmHg, azotemia (serum creatinine >1.5)
Dose	Start with Captopril 6.25 mg p.o. b.i.d. and monitor blood pressure Increase to 12.5 mg b.i.d., then 25 mg b.i.d. or until systolic blood pressure falls slightly Avoid dropping systolic blood pressure below 110 mmHg
Timing	Start 2–3 days after acute MI; continue indefinitely
Potential benefits	Reduction of afterload may prevent infarct expansion and LV dilatation in patients with large MI

be noted that these studies were performed with patients who were not treated with thrombolytic agents. Pfeffer's study of anterior infarction found that the beneficial effects of captopril were limited to patients with persistent occlusion of the infarct artery. Similar trials in patients who have had thrombolytic therapy are needed, but in the meantime we are recommending long-term ACE inhibitor therapy for patients with large MI (ejection fraction <45% at hospital discharge, Table 8.6).

Summary and recommendations

Our current recommendations are based upon incomplete data. Many of the adjunctive therapies have been studied in patients with acute MI, but there have been few studies in patients with MI plus thrombolytic therapy. Presently, we recommend aspirin and intravenous heparin therapy for all patients (although there remains controversy about intravenous heparin). With no contraindication, we use beta blockers. Intravenous nitroglycerin may be useful in patients with uncontrolled hypertension or, when used cautiously, for those with CHF (high preload). The routine use of intravenous nitroglycerin to prevent coronary spasm and therefore reocclusion has not been proven. You must remember that nitroglycerin had deleterious effects on LV function when it caused hypotension (systolic pressure below 100 mmHg). Calcium channel blockers have not been found to have definite benefit acutely, but may be useful for patients with "incomplete" infarction who have residual stenosis of the infarct artery and who will not be having revascularization. Acute use of ACE inhibitors is not indicated, but long-term therapy with captopril is recommended for patients with MI and LVEF <45%.

It is a long list of drugs. What do you use for a given patient? The clinical situation often helps us make the decision. Let us consider recently treated patients.

Patient 1

A 56-year-old man with anterior infarction and a history of obstructive lung disease had anterior MI and was treated within 3 hours with intravenous STK: definitely treat with aspirin and heparin. Because of the lung disease we would avoid beta blocker therapy. If systolic blood pressure is above 120 mmHg, we would add intravenous nitroglycerin at 5 μg per minute and titrate the dose until systolic blood pressure is lowered to 100–110 mmHg (Table 8.4). If serum magnesium is low, we would add intravenous magnesium sulfate (Table 8.5). As nitrates are being given to lower blood pressure, we would not use calcium blockers as well. If an echocardiogram or nuclear study shows below 45%, treat with captopril (Table 8.6).

Patient 2

A 70-year-old woman with acute inferior MI treated with rt-PA and with a past history of hypertension: definitely treat with aspirin and heparin. With elevated blood pressure in the absence of bradyarrhythmia or wheezing, we would also treat with intravenous metropolol or atenolol (Table 8.3). If blood pressure remains elevated we would add intravenous nitroglycerin as described above. Because she has been hypertensive and possibly treated with thiazide diuretics, we would pay particular attention to serum magnesium and replace any deficit. If she (or any other patient) refuses angiography or revascularization we would consider long-term therapy with calcium channel blockers and beta blockers.

Patient 3

A 38-year-old man with acute anterior infarction treated at 4 hours with rt-PA has systolic blood pressure 80 mmHg, bibasilar rales, and low urine output: definitely treat with aspirin and heparin. His low blood pressure excludes use of beta blockers or intravenous nitroglycerin. We would replace serum magnesium if his level is low, especially as he is at high risk for malignant arrhythmias with his large and complicated infarction. Watch for further drop in blood pressure with intravenous magnesium sulfate (Table 8.5). With borderline shock we would also consider urgent angiography and emergency angioplasty if the infarct artery remains closed. Because of hypotension, calcium blockers would not be used. Long-term captopril therapy may be appropriate if LVEF is <45% and systolic blood pressure is above 100 mmHg; it should be started 2–3 days after MI.

Patient 4

A 52-year-old man with acute inferior infarction treated at 4 hours with rt-PA; at the time of initial evaluation he has intermittent Wenckebach phenomenon and a ventricular rate of 45/minute, and a systolic blood pressure of 80 mmHg: definitely treat with aspirin and heparin. If he has no pulmonary congestion, consider a fluid challenge. He is not a candidate for beta blocker therapy because of the bradyarrhythmia. We would not use intravenous nitroglycerin because of the low blood pressure. (If systolic blood pressure was above 110 mmHg, intravenous nitroglycerin would be a good choice.) If the slow heart rate appears responsible for his hypotension it may respond to atropine and may even require temporary pacing. If calcium blocker therapy is to be used after thrombolysis, choose an agent less likely to aggravate AV nodal block, such as nifedipine. But do not rush into pacemaker therapy as thrombolysis may lead to prompt resolution of the bradyarrhythmia (Fig. 6.3).

Selected reading

Becker RC, Gore JM. Adjunctive use of beta-adrenergic blockers, calcium antagonists and other therapies in coronary thrombolysis. Am J Cardiol 1991;67:25–31A.

Chesebro JH, Fuster V. Dynamic thrombosis and thrombolysis. Circulation 1991; 83:1815–17.

Eisenberg PR. Role of new anticoagulants as adjunctive therapy during thrombolysis. Am J Cardiol 1991;67:19–24A.

Gibson RS, Boden WE, Theroux P, *et al*. Diltiazem and reinfarction in patients with non-Q-wave myocardial infarction. N Engl J Med 1986; 315:423–29.

ISIS-1 Collaborative Group. Randomised trial of intravenous atenolol among 16 027 cases of suspected acute myocardial infarction: ISIS-1. Lancet 1986;2:57–66.

Jugdutt BI, Sussex BA, Tymchak WJ, Warnica JW. Intravenous nitroglycerin in the early management of acute myocardial infarction. Cardiovasc Rev Rep 1989;10:29–35.

Jugdutt BI, Warnica JW. Intravenous nitroglycerin therapy to limit myocardial infarct size, expansion, and complications. Effect of timing, dosage, and infarct location. Circulation 1988;78:906.

The Miami Trial Research Group. MIAMI. A randomised placebo-controlled international trial. Eur Heart J 1985;6:199–226.

Multicenter Diltiazem Postinfarction Trial Research Group. The effect of diltiazem on mortality and reinfarction after myocardial infarction. New Engl J Med 1988;319:385–92.

Pfeffer MA, Lamas GA, Vaughan DE, Parisi AF, Braunwald E. Effect of captopril on progressive ventricular dilatation after anterior myocardial infarction. N Engl J Med 1988;319:80–6.

Popma JJ, Topol EJ. Adjuncts to thrombolysis for myocardial reperfusion. Ann Int Med 1991;115:34–44.

Prins MH, Hirsh J. Heparin as an adjunctive treatment after thrombolytic therapy for acute myocardial infarction. Am J Cardiol 1991;67:3–11A.

Sharpe N, Smith H, Murphy J, Hannan S. Treatment of patients with symptomless left ventricular dysfunction after myocardial infarction. Lancet 1988;1:255–59.

Willerson JT, Buja LM. Protection of the myocardium during myocardial infarction: Pharmacologic protection during thrombolytic therapy. Am J Cardiol 1990;65:35I–41I.

Yusuf S, Sleight P, Held P, McMahon S. Routine medical management of acute myocardial infarction. Circulation 1990;82(Suppl II):117–34.

Yusuf S, Peto R, Lewis J, Collins R, Sleight P. Beta blockade during and after myocardial infarction: An overview of the randomized trials. Prog Cardiovasc Dis 1985;27:335–71.

Yusuf S, Held P, Furberg C. Update of effects of calcium antagonists in myocardial infarction or angina in light of the second Danish verapamil infarction trial (DAVIT-II) and other recent studies. Am J Cardiol 1991;67:1295–97.

Yusuf S, MacMahon S, Collins R, Peto R. Effect of intravenous nitrates on mortality in acute myocardial infarction: An overview of the randomised trials. Lancet 1988;1:1088–92.

Chapter 9
Complications of thrombolytic therapy

Bleeding

The thrombolytic system is unable to distinguish between hemostatic plug at the site of vessel injury and pathological, occlusive thrombus in a coronary artery (Fig. 4.1). Disruption of the hemostatic plug will cause bleeding. When describing thrombolytic therapy to the patient and his or her family, it is important to emphasize that these drugs "dissolve blood clot," that clinically significant bleeding occurs in 5–10% of patients, and that bleeding can be serious, requiring blood transfusion in 2–3% of patients.

Each of the thrombolytic drugs carries an equivalent and substantial risk of bleeding. Theoretically, more extensive fibrinogenolysis with STK and APSAC would increase the risk of bleeding, but most studies have found that the risk of bleeding is not proportional to the degree of fibrinogen depletion. Comparative drug trials, including CITTS, which compared STK and rt-PA, have found a similar incidence of bleeding for all of the available thrombolytic agents.

Bleeding does not develop spontaneously in patients with normal, intact vasculature. Instead, bleeding appears related to identifiable pathology: an arterial puncture site, stress ulceration, gastritis, kidney stone, bladder polyp or tumor, colonic polyp, etc. Patients who develop bleeding after thrombolytic therapy or during anticoagulant therapy should be evaluated for specific pathology that may have caused the bleeding. This underscores the importance of screening patients for potential sources of bleeding before thrombolytic therapy. When there is no clear contraindication to treatment but the patient appears to have a somewhat higher risk of bleeding, take all appropriate prophylactic measures. For example, if there is a remote history of ulcer disease, do not hesitate to treat with antacids, H2 blockers, and/or sucralfate.

Table 9.1 Complications — community hospitals and the tertiary referral center (From Taylor, et al. J Am Board Fam Pract 1990;3:1–6. Complications were reported only when intervention was required i.e., stopping or changing a drug, addition of new therapy, special diagnostic procedures)

	Community hospital ($n = 816$)	Referral center ($n = 196$)
Bleeding site		
Total bleeds	82 (10.1%)	26 (13.3%)
Transfusion	17 (2.1%)	7 (3.6%)
GI bleed	30 (3.7%)	7 (3.6%)
Transfusion	12 (1.5%)	1 (0.5%)
GU bleed	12 (1.5%)	0
Transfusion	0	0
CNS bleed	2 (0.3%)	1 (0.5%)
Transfusion	0	0
Cath. site bleed	22 (2.7%)	16 (8.2%)
Transfusion	2 (0.3%)	5 (2.6%)
Other bleeds	16 (2.0%)	2 (1.0%)
Transfusion	3 (0.4%)	1 (0.5%)
Allergic reaction (anaphylaxis)	0	0
Death	39 (5%)	12 (6%)

Risk of bleeding

We prospectively collected data from 1012 patients who were treated with intravenous STK from 1982 through 1987. From 1988–90 the CITTS was done randomly, comparing STK and rt-PA in 253 patients. Tables 9.1 and 9.2 outline complications from these two trials. In the large observational trial of 1012 patients we compared patients treated in community hospitals with those treated in the referral center, and found that the incidence of complications (and the success rate as measured by an open infarct artery) was no different for patients treated by primary care physicians in community hospitals. CITTS also found no difference in complication rates when comparing rt-PA and STK, and this has been the experience of other trials which compared different agents. The incidence of bleeding in these two studies is similar to that described by other large trials.

Table 9.2 Complications — CITTS. (Taylor *et al.*) Complications were reported only when intervention was required (i.e., stopping or changing a drug, addition of new therapy, special diagnostic procedures)

	STK (*n* = 130)	rt-PA (*n* = 123)	*p* value
*Bleeding site**			
GI bleed	6 (5%)	4 (3%)	NS
Transfusions	2 (1.5%)	1 (0.8%)	
GU bleed	3 (2%)	0	
Transfusions	0	0	
CNS bleed	1 (0.7%)	2 (1.6%)	
Cath site bleed	13 (10%)	10 (8%)	
Transfusions	1 (0.7%)	2 (1.6%)	
Venipunctures	2 (1.5%)	2 (1.6%)	
Transfusions	2 (1.5%)	0	
Any bleed	36 (28%)	26 (21%)	
Transfusions	4 (3%)	3 (2%)	
Embolic stroke	1 (0.7%)	1 (0.7%)	
Allergic reaction			
Anaphylaxis	0	0	
Rash	3 (2%)	0	
Death	9 (6.9%)	6 (4.9%)	

CNS, central nervous system.

Hematoma

Our treatment strategy included early angiography, within 48 hours of thrombolytic therapy. As with similar studies that included early catheterization, hematoma at the catheterization site was our most common bleeding complication. Hematoma occurred more commonly in elderly patients, especially women. Only two of the 1265 patients in these two studies required surgical drainage of a groin hematoma and arterial repair. Although groin hematoma can be an aggravating problem following thrombolysis, we do not consider it a serious enough problem to warrant avoiding early angiography. In fact, we and most others find it unnecessary to alter heparin therapy before angiography.

We are especially careful with arterial puncture technique, and routinely canulate the vessel using a 1-wall stick. We also use the smallest diagnostic catheter system that will work, 6 French catheters for large patients and 5 French catheters for small patients. If the patient is within 24 hours of thrombolytic therapy an arterial line is left in place until the next day. The catheter is removed only if activated partial thromboplastin time, prothrombin time, and platelet count are normal. If there is uncertainty, we also check the fibrinogen level. More recently, we have been monitoring activated clotting time in the catheterization laboratory before pulling arterial lines.

Despite these precautions, we have learned that catheterization site hematoma may develop if we puncture an artery 24–48 hours after thrombolytic therapy. How much worse would it be if an artery is punctured at the time of thrombolytic therapy? Unfortunately, we have the opportunity to answer this question intermittently with patients who have had "routine" arterial blood gases drawn at the time of presentation to their emergency department. Hematoma in the anticubital fossa after arterial blood gases are some of the worse bleeds that we have encountered after thrombolytic therapy. We have had elderly patients who have required transfusion, and who have spent many extra days in hospital with their arms elevated. One patient had compression injury of the median nerve. We have had no patient lose an arm, but it seems that we have come close.

There is *no need* for routine arterial blood gases at the time of acute MI. You may consider blood gases for patients with impending respiratory failure or with a history of serious obstructive lung disease. But patients with mild respiratory distress, even with a history of prior lung disease, can be managed without arterial gases. Our emergency department and CCU nurses routinely place a sign above the patient's bed warning laboratory personnel to avoid arterial sticks (Fig. 9.1).

Older patients and women appear more susceptible to hematoma after arterial puncture. This is the case with venipuncture as well. These patients often develop extensive hematoma at i.v. sites. Many of these can be avoided if nursing and laboratory staffs understand the need for special attention to hemostasis. Pressure dressing over a venipuncture site should be considered for patients who have had recent thrombolytic therapy. It is important to check *under* all pressure dressings for developing hematoma.

Older patients with fragile skin may develop an apparently spontaneous hematoma in other areas. We have seen older

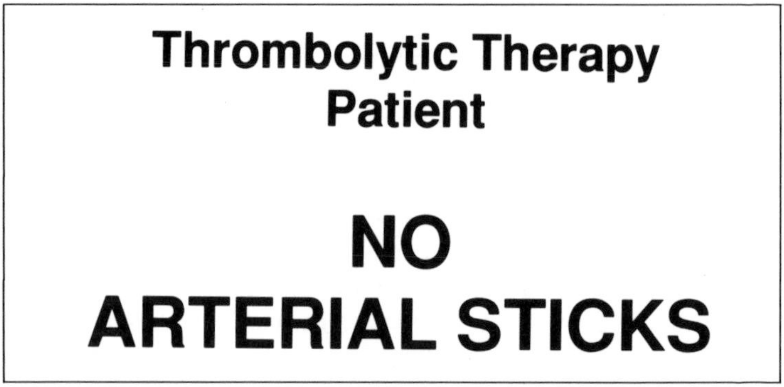

Fig. 9.1 Our nurses place this sign near patients who have had thrombolytic therapy.

patients develop a hematoma over the buttocks and back related to bedrest. Others have had hematoma develop under the blood pressure cuff. Use of automatic sphygmomanometers may cause more bruising and require special caution. All patients should be handled gently after thrombolytic therapy, but especially the elderly.

GI bleeding
Significant GI bleeding accounted for the largest proportion of "significant" bleeds, those requiring transfusion. In our series we classified any GI specimen that was hemoccult positive as a GI bleed. Most were easily controlled by stopping the thrombolytic drug or heparin and treating with antacids, H2 blockers, and sucralfate. With more serious GI bleeds we routinely get consultation from a gastroenterologist. Endoscopy reveals the same variety of pathology that causes GI bleeding in other clinical settings (gastritis, ulcers, Mallory-Weiss tears, colonic polyps, and tumors, etc.). We had one patient with serious bleeding from esophageal varices who denied his alcohol history at the time of initial evaluation. Although transfusion has been required on multiple occasions, we have had no patient die because of GI bleeding. One patient required emergency surgery to control bleeding resulting from a perforated ulcer.

GI bleeding occurred more commonly 1–5 days after thrombolytic therapy while the patient was on heparin. It was less frequently seen during the administration of the thrombolytic agent. This was true of other bleeding complications of thrombolytic therapy as well. Stress ulceration may occur more commonly in critically ill patients. We do not hesitate to treat our sickest patients with prophylactic H2 blockers. With any history to suggest higher risk of GI bleeding we add sucralfate (Carafate®).

Other bleeding complications

Bleeding from other sites is also possible and is commonly related to specific pathology. Patients with a history of kidney stones are more prone to developing hematuria. When hematuria is mild we continue anticoagulant therapy. If the rate of bleeding increases, heparin is stopped. It is rare for these patients to require transfusion (Tables 9.1, 9.2). Because of the high probability of urinary tract pathology, urological evaluation should be considered during the next few weeks. It is useful to have expert help, and we have a low threshhold for requesting urology consultation. As an example, a recent patient had urethral injury when urinary catheter insertion was difficult at the time of acute MI. We were alarmed by the amount of bleeding, but the urologist was not. He placed an indwelling catheter without difficulty, and local pressure from the catheter controlled bleeding. He advised us to continue heparin therapy. The catheter was removed 6 days later without recurrence of bleeding.

It is common to have a substantial drop in hemoglobin and hematocrit when patients have bleeding. Even without apparent bleeding patients may drop hemoglobin 1–2 g during the week after thrombolytic therapy. Careful examination of such patients usually reveals hematoma at a venipuncture site or elsewhere that are larger than expected. When there is a more substantial drop in hemoglobin it is usually caused from an occult bleeding source. Bleeding into the retroperitoneal space should be considered. We have seen patients with deep hematoma in the thigh or buttock that lowered hemoglobin by 2–4 g and that were not clinically obvious on examination for a couple of days. Another patient had active bleeding into the rectus abdominus muscle which persisted for 5 days with only mild abdominal discomfort. The diagnosis finally was made with a CT scan of the abdomen. Serious bleeding from the GI or genito-urinary tracts usually is obvious and rarely occult.

Management of bleeding

The hemostatic defect

A patient with recent thrombolytic therapy who is on heparin and daily aspirin has a number of different hemostatic defects. Among these is the active fibrinolytic state as described in Chapter 4. The active lytic state occurs when there is free plasmin in the circulation. Plasmin digests fibrin, but also digests fibrinogen and other clotting factors (Fig. 4.1). This depletion of clotting factors, fibrinogen, and factors V and VIII, represents another serious hemostatic defect. Fibrin degradation products contribute another, and the antithrombin action of heparin therapy adds to defective hemostasis as well.

Aspirin therapy causes permanent dysfunction of platelets. Correction requires replacement of the defective platelets. Since the half-life of platelets is 4 days, normalization of the bleeding time may be delayed 3–6 days after stopping aspirin. The effects of other antiplatelet agents such as dipyridamole are reversible when therapy is discontinued. Other drugs with antiplatelet activity include intravenous nitroglycerin, calcium antagonists, angiographic contrast agents, and beta blockers.

Laboratory studies

There are a number of laboratory tests that are helpful in monitoring patients who are bleeding following thrombolysis, and they are directly related to the hemostatic defects catalogued above. Activated partial thromboplastin time and thrombin time are guides not only to the effect of heparin, but also to identify a persistent lytic state in the absence of heparin. The *fibrinogen level* is especially important. Patients usually stop bleeding when fibrinogen has been replaced to a level of 1 g/liter. Bleeding time is a measure of platelet function and is useful when considering patients for platelet transfusion. It is possible to specifically measure clotting factors V and VIII, and to measure $alpha_2$–antiplasmin, but these tests are not readily available in most hospitals. Fibrin degradation products indicate an active lytic state, but measurement takes time and the result usually returns too late to influence clinical decisions.

In fact, the initial decision to replace clotting factors in patients with life-threatening hemorrhage is usually empirical, and laboratory studies are more useful as a guide to subsequent steps.

General measures/transfusion

General principles for management of bleeding apply. Good intravenous access must be secured. Patients who are actively lytic should not have subclavian lines (do not compound the problem). We consider transfusion for patients with hematocrit <30% who have active, severe bleeding. As these patients also have active ischemic heart disease and recent MI, it is especially important to stay ahead of the bleeding if possible. Stop heparin and anti-platelet drugs, and draw blood for platelet count, aPTT, prothrombin time, and fibrinogen level.

Cryoprecipitate

Cryoprecipitate contains fibrinogen and factor VIII. Ten units of cryoprecipitate raises the fibrinogen level about 0.7 g/liter and raises factor VIII to an effective level; this dose is adequate for most patients. If the follow-up fibrinogen level is lower than 1.0 g/liter, another 10 unit dose should be given. As cryoprecipitate is a pooled blood product there is risk of transfusion related infection. The risk of AIDS for each unit of cryoprecipitate is the same as that for a single unit of blood. Following replacement therapy, fibrinogen has a half-life of 3–4 days and factor VIII, 9–18 hours. If there is active thrombolysis, both will be depleted faster.

Fresh frozen plasma (FFP)

FFP also contains factor VIII but contains factor V and alpha$_2$-antiplasmin as well (Chapter 4). FFP must be infused quickly as both factors V and VIII are labile. The half-life of factor V is 15–36 hours. Full replacement of factor V with FFP is not necessary as platelet transfusions also contain substantial quantities of factor V.

Platelet transfusion

Platelet packs contain about 50 ml plasma and thus provide factors V and VIII as well as platelets. In addition, platelets themselves contribute almost 25% of the factor V found in whole blood. A bleeding time and platelet count should be measured before platelet transfusion. But if bleeding is catastrophic, give platelet transfusions immediately. The platelet count may be misleading. With recent aspirin therapy the platelet count may be adequate but the platelets may be dysfunctional. Do not hesitate to give platelet transfusion despite an adequate platelet count in patients recently treated with aspirin (in this situation bleeding time will be prolonged).

Antifibrinolytic drugs

The antifibrinolytic agents inhibit plasminogen activators and block the effects of circulating plasmin; the lytic state produced by any of the thrombolytic agents is reversed. All of the activators of the fibrinolytic system work to produce plasmin. The anti-fibrinolytic agents work by inhibiting the binding of plasmin to fibrin, and to inhibit the binding of plasminogen to circulating fibrinogen. They also may inhibit binding of rt-PA to fibrin.

Antifibrinolytic agents are not required for most patients with bleeding after thrombolytic therapy. Most episodes of bleeding occur after the lytic state has passed, while patients are on anti-coagulants or have depletion of clotting factors. Replacement of clotting factors is adequate therapy. Antifibrinolytic drugs should be considered for patients who have life-threatening bleeding which occurs near the time of thrombolytic therapy, during the lytic phase. Laboratory studies which suggest an active lytic phase include prolonged aPTT or prolonged thrombin time (in the absence of heparin therapy), and elevated fibrin degradation products. But do not wait for these test results to tell you when to use antifibrinolytic drugs. It is a clinical decision. If the patient is within *12 hours* of receiving the thrombolytic drug (particularly APSAC), and has life-threatening bleeding, consider anti-fibrinolytic therapy.

There are good reasons to avoid antifibrinolytic agents if at all possible. As soon as the agents are given, fibrinolysis stops. Furthermore, the antifibrinolytic drugs are bound to the thrombus and make the thrombus resistant to further thrombolytic therapy. Recall that thrombolytic therapy also activates clotting factors and platelets producing a paradoxical, prothrombotic state. In a sense, there is an equilibrium between thrombosis and throm-bolysis. Abruptly halting fibrinolysis exposes the patient to unopposed thrombosis. Rethrombosis of the coronary artery is likely. If the patient is having urological bleeding, abrupt throm-bosis and ureteral obstruction may occur.

Two antifibrinolytic drugs are available, aminocaproic acid and tranexamic acid. Aminocaproic acid has been the agent of choice, probably because of its shorter half-life (Table 9.3), and because our hospital pharmacy does not stock tranexamic acid. A loading dose of 5 g of aminocaproic acid is given intravenously over 30–60 minutes, and then 0.5–1 g per hour by continuous infusion. Plasma half-life is 1–2 hours with total duration of antifibrinolytic effect <3 hours. An important contraindication to the use of aminocaproic acid is disseminated intravascular coagulation (DIC) which is aggravated by the drug. This may seem a rare possibility, but patients with large infarction and

Table 9.3 Antifibrinolytic therapy

	Aminocaproic acid
Indications	Major bleeding with 12 hours of thrombolytic therapy (during the "lytic" phase)
Mechanisms	Inhibits plasminogen activation Blocks binding of plasmin to fibrin
Half-life	1–2 hours
Dose	5 g i.v. over 30–60 min 0.5–1.0 g/h i.v. infusion
Duration of effect	<3 hours
Contraindications	DIC
Cautions	May provoke thrombosis: Coronary rethrombosis is possible Use with caution for urological bleeding

shock may be at risk for developing DIC. When patients are this complicated, consultative help from the hematology and laboratory medicine services is critical.

Protamine sulfate

Because of the short half-life of heparin, most patients with bleeding can be managed without reversing it with protamine sulfate. Use protamine for the patient who has been on continuous infusion of heparin within the last 4 hours or who has just received a large bolus infusion. To reverse the effects of a bolus infusion of heparin, give 1 mg of protamine sulfate for every 100 U heparin (for instance, a 5000 unit bolus of heparin is reversed by 50 mg protamine sulfate). Thirty minutes later you need only half that dose of protamine. For a patient who is on a continuous heparin infusion, calculate the total dose of heparin received during the previous 4 hours and give 1 mg protamine sulfate for each 100 U heparin. (Thus, 1200 U per hour × 4 hours equals 4800 U heparin; give 48 mg protamine sulfate.) Infuse protamine slowly, over 10 minutes.

Protamine is a fish product. We have used it commonly in the cardiac catheterization laboratory, and we have learned to ask patients about fish allergy before giving the drug. Rashes and hives are common after administering protamine, and anaphylaxis is a possibility. Patients with a fish allergy are usually given an intravenous antihistamine (Benadryl® 50 mg i.v.) before protamine. Previous exposure to protamine also increases the risk of allergic reaction; this includes diabetic patients using protamine zinc insulin.

Intracranial hemorrhage

Intracranial bleeding is observed in 0.3–1.6% of patients treated with thrombolytic agents (Tables 9.1, 9.2). The risk of intracranial bleeding is higher for elderly patients and those with a history of poorly controlled hypertension. History of stroke may increase the risk of intracranial bleeding, and any head trauma clearly does.

The risk of intracranial hemorrhage may be higher with rt-PA than with other thrombolytic agents. The ISIS-3 trial noted probable intracranial bleeding in 0.5% of patients treated with STK and 0.7% of those treated with rt-PA, and this difference was statistically significant because of the large number of patients studied. There are a few ways to look at these numbers. You could say that bleeding was 40% more common with rt-PA (0.2% ÷ 0.5%), 28% less common with STK (0.2% ÷ 0.7%), or that the risk of bleeding with rt-PA might affect two more patients per 1000 treated (seven rather than five per 1000). While the result was statistically significant, the risk of bleeding with each of the agents is low and the absolute difference between the two drugs is small (Figs 9.2, 9.3).

Intracranial hemorrhage is a devastating complication. During our 10-year experience, the only death we can directly relate to a complication of a thrombolytic agent was a patient who died with intracranial bleeding. It is important to look for warning signs before thrombolytic therapy. One of our patients had fallen and bumped his head prior to arrival in the emergency department. Because of his chest pain and the excitement of the moment he forgot to mention it. In retrospect there was a small contusion over one eye that was missed at the time of initial examination. Two days later he appeared lethargic, but with no other neurological symptoms. A CT scan confirmed frontal lobe hematoma. In addition to careful history we have learned that specifically examining the head for evidence of injury is worthwhile (perhaps as useful as the cardiac examination).

Intracranial hemorrhage plays a role in the ongoing controversy

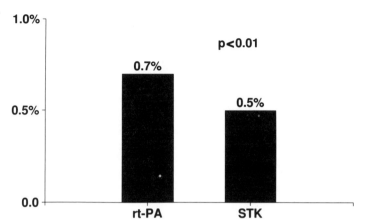

Fig. 9.2 There are a couple of ways to interpret the intracranial bleeding rate in the ISIS-3 study. In this figure there is a 40% higher bleeding rate with rt-PA. This is a dramatic result.

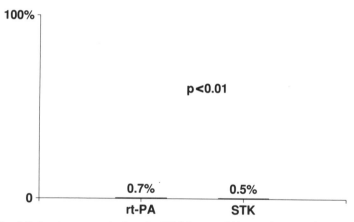

Fig. 9.3 Another way to look at the ISIS-3 intracranial hemorrhage rate is to present the absolute risk of bleeding for patients. There is still a 40% higher risk of bleeding with rt-PA, but the real risk which each patient faces before therapy is obviously quite low, regardless of which thrombolytic agent is used. On this and Figure 9.2, the intracranial bleeding rate of APSAC, 0.6%, is not included.

about heparin after thrombolytic therapy. Full dose, intravenous heparin therapy probably increases the risk of intracranial hemorrhage. The ISIS-3 trial used subcutaneous heparin for most patients, and the intracranial bleeding rate ranged from 0.5–0.7% for the three drugs. A small subset of patients in this trial was treated with full dose intravenous heparin. This was not done by study design but instead by physician preference; most of the patients in this international study who received intravenous heparin were treated in the United States. The intracranial bleeding rate was much higher for these patients. The ISIS-3 investigators are reluctant to draw conclusions as these data did not come from the formal trial. But because of this information, the ongoing GUSTO study will directly compare subcutaneous and intravenous heparin in a group of patients treated with STK.

Cardiac complications of thrombolytic therapy

Death from LV failure, cardiogenic shock, or cardiac arrhythmias are complications of acute MI, but not of thrombolytic therapy. These negative outcomes have occurred more commonly in patients treated with placebo than with thrombolytic agents in the large, randomized trials. As discussed in Chapter 6 reperfusion arrhythmia is a rare cause of death, and VF occurs more commonly in placebo-treated patients.

Cardiac rupture

Cardiac rupture is one complication of MI that may be increased with thrombolytic agents. It has been reported in 3–4% of patients with acute MI. But it may be more common in patients after thrombolytic therapy. Autopsy studies of patients who died in clinical trials of thrombolytic therapy identified cardiac rupture in as many as 38%. It is possible that hemorrhage into areas of infarction is more common after thrombolytic therapy. Intramural bleeding may cause dissection along planes of necrotic tissue, then myocardial rupture. Timing of thrombolytic therapy may be important. Transmural necrosis may be prevented in patients who have thrombolysis early in the course of infarction. Necrosis would be more prevalent in patients treated later. Honan *et al.*, 1990, analyzed data from multiple studies involving over 44 000 patients. They found that thrombolytic therapy *early* in the course of infarction reduced overall mortality rates and also reduced the risk of myocardial rupture. But they found that treatment of patients beyond 11 hours after onset of symptoms increases the risk of rupture. Interestingly, overall mortality was beneficially effected by treatment within 21 hours. They suggest that patients treated from 11–21 hours have an overall improved mortality risk, but a higher risk of death from cardiac rupture. Beyond 21 hours there was no overall mortality benefit, and the risk of rupture was even higher. They are careful to point out that the methods of this study are imprecise. We do not feel that these time limits should be used to govern therapy for the individual patient. On the other hand we agree with the general message: later therapy increases the risk of myocardial rupture.

It is noteworthy that beta blocker therapy may lower the risk of myocardial rupture by reducing blood pressure and contractility and thus lower the wall tension. We would favor the use of beta blockers as adjunctive therapy for patients who are treated late in the course of MI, especially those with elevated blood pressure (Table 8.3).

Allergic reaction

Allergic reactions may occur with both STK and APSAC, and are not seen with rt-PA and UK (both native proteins). The most common allergic reactions are mild and include rash, angioneurotic edema, or flushing. Life-threatening anaphylactic shock is rare, occurring in fewer than 1 in 1000 patients. In earlier days severe allergic reactions to STK were more common as the drug preparation was impure. The manufacturing process has changed and the STK available today is relatively pure. The incidence of serious allergic reactions reported in the older literature no longer applies.

Both STK and APSAC illicit antibody response which begins in 4–6 days, peaks in several weeks, and returns to baseline about 6 months later. Antibody levels vary from patient to patient. Recall that these antibodies will "neutralize" STK that is infused and thus reduce effectiveness of STK. For this reason, and because of the potential for allergic reactions, repeat treatment with both STK and APSAC is avoided for 6 months after initial therapy. If MI recurs patients should be treated with rt-PA.

Management of mild allergic reactions includes antihistamine and steroid administration. There is no need to pretreat patients before using STK or APSAC, or to use a test dose.

Hypotension

Hypotension is seen with all the thrombolytic agents, but more commonly with APSAC and STK. The large ISIS-3 study described hypotension in 4.3% of patients treated with rt-PA compared with 6.8% treated with STK. APSAC caused hypotension more commonly than both STK and rt-PA. In the CITTS trials, hypotension rarely prevented administration of the full dose of STK. We treat hypotension by reducing the infusion rate of the thrombolytic drug and with volume expansion using normal saline.

Selected readings

Honan MB, Harrell FE, Reimer KA, *et al.* Cardiac rupture, mortality and the timing of thrombolytic therapy: A meta-analysis. J Am Coll Cardiol 1990;16:359–67.

ISIS-3. Presented at the annual meeting of the American College of Cardiology, Atlanta, Georgia, March 1991.

Sherry S. Bleeding complications in thrombolytic therapy. Hosp Pract 1990;25(Suppl 5):1–21.

Taylor GJ, Moses HW, Koester DL, *et al.* Comparison of intravenous tissue plasminogen activator (rt-PA) and streptokinase therapy for acute ST-segment elevation myocardial infarction: Improved regional wall motion in patients with anterior infarction treated with rt-PA. The Central Illinois Thrombolytic Therapy Study (CITTS) (Unpublished data).

Taylor GJ, Song A, Moses HW, *et al.* The primary care physician and thrombolytic therapy for acute myocardial infarction: Comparison of intravenous streptokinase in community hospitals and the tertiary referral center. J Am Board Fam Pract 1990;3:1–6.

Chapter 10
Rapid application

Time means muscle. Every trial that has examined time to thrombolytic therapy and efficacy has found that the patients treated earliest have the best clinical result. GISSI-1 found an 18% decrease in mortality for patients treated with STK. Those who were treated within 3 hours had a 23% decrease in mortality, and those treated 3–6 hours after onset of pain, had a 17% decrease. After 6 hours, no survival benefit was found in this study (although ISIS-2 showed improved survival in patients treated after 6–12 hours). A small group in the GISSI-1 trial was treated within 1 hour of onset of pain, and they had a 47% reduction in mortality.

We believe that anything you do to hasten the opening of the infarct artery by 30 minutes will produce a significant clinical benefit for your patient. "Faster" drugs provide one approach. But it makes little sense to find a drug that is 30 minutes faster if you and your emergency department are 1 hour too slow.

How long does it take you to give thrombolytic therapy in your emergency department? When we asked ourselves that question 2–3 years ago our immediate response was "30 minutes." And "30 minutes" is the answer we get from most programs. But we have been fooling ourselves. When we retrospectively examined emergency department records we found that average time to therapy was 84 minutes. This was not because we were inexperienced. On the contrary, we had been treating patients with acute MI with thrombolytic therapy for 7 years when we did this survey. A national survey of experienced hospitals also found that the average delay from arrival in the emergency department to thrombolytic therapy was 1 hour and 30 minutes. That is an appalling result.

We set out to improve our record, and after a major effort have cut the time to therapy to 34 minutes in our emergency department (Moses, *et al.*, 1991). This was more difficult to accomplish than most of our doctors and nurses anticipated. Although every-

Table 10.1 Key steps in reducing time to treatment with thrombolytic therapy

Rapid triage
Immediate ECG
Treat in the emergency department
Standardized orders
Two nurses
The first doctor treats
Brief informed consent
Drugs in emergency department
No routine chest X-ray
Single laboratory request
No routine blood gases
Do not wait for laboratory results
Two i.v. lines initially
Play the odds
Poster in emergency department
Involve the staff

one involved agreed with the goal, it took us a full year to implement the changes outlined in this chapter. Practice patterns are difficult to change. The most important step was establishing a committee of physicians and nurses whose responsibility was to effect these changes. This committee carried the authority of the medical staff. It continues to meet periodically to assess management of patients with chest pain in the emergency department.

Changes that improved time to treatment

The key elements of our new rapid treatment protocol are summarized in Table 10.1.

Rapid triage of patients with suspected MI is essential. Any patient with chest pain must get top priority and be moved to a special section of the emergency department and placed on a monitor. One i.v. line should be started while doing the ECG and getting a history.

The critical step seems to be getting an immediate ECG. Our goal is that every patient with chest pain must have an ECG within 5 minutes of arrival in the emergency department. In our hospital, an ECG machine was not routinely kept in the emergency department. We now have one in the emergency department at all times, and all emergency department nurses and technicians are trained to do an ECG. If you use a computerized ECG reading system, there should be no delay because of computerization. Do not wait for the computer interpretation. The emergency department physician must be able to make a diagnosis based upon his or her own reading of the ECG. Computer readings often are erroneous, and you cannot wait for the corrected reading.

Treat the patient in the emergency department and not after transfer to the CCU. A surprising number of hospitals persist in transferring the patient to the CCU before treatment is given. Doctors invariably comment that it "takes little time to transfer the patient, and our CCU nurses are the ones used to giving thrombolytic drugs." But this inexcuseably delays treatment. No matter how slick your system is, there will be times when a bed will not be ready, and the patient will wait in the emergency department another 30 minutes. (This is usually the case in our hospital.) When the patient finally arrives in the CCU the nurse taking care of him or her will have to get report and do a brief clinical evaluation before starting the thrombolytic drug. The correct place to start thrombolytic therapy is the emergency department, and the emergency department nurses naturally will become the most experienced in the hospital in using these drugs.

Two nurses should attend the patient with chest pain. A lot must be done quickly (drawing laboratory work, starting i.v.s, getting the ECG, hooking up the monitor, vital signs . . .). At least two pairs of hands are needed. If the hospital is a small one with limited emergency department staff, we suggest routinely having a CCU nurse come to the emergency department to help with the patient. It will be faster for the CCU nurse to come to the patient than for the patient to go to the CCU.

Thrombolytic therapy must be ordered by the physician who evaluates the patient first. If you are uncomfortable with this, perhaps you should not place yourself in a setting where you must treat patients with acute MI. Referral to a cardiologist causes inappropriate delay. Our medical staff also has decided that thrombolytic therapy should not be delayed in order to notify the primary care physician. Our emergency department doctors treat the patient, then call the primary care physician. It is the responsibility of the emergency department physician to promptly treat other life-threatening conditions; acute MI is no different.

Informed consent is important, and explaining the need for treatment and haste does not substantially delay therapy. As discussed in Chapter 5, we are split on whether or not to have patients sign a consent form. As there is morbidity and mortality with MI and thrombolytic therapy, having the patient and his or her family give written consent is reasonable but not mandatory. The consent form we currently use is reproduced as Table 5.1.

The commonly used thrombolytic agents should be stored in the emergency department for rapid mixing and administration. There should not be a delay because of transfer of these drugs from the pharmacy.

The chest X-ray usually should be done after the decision about thrombolytic therapy has been made and thrombolytic therapy has been started. If there is uncertainty about the diagnosis of acute MI because of an equivocal ECG or history, the chest X-ray may be useful. For example, dissecting aortic aneurysm may cause widening of the mediastinum on chest X-ray. In addition, pneumonia or pneumothorax both can cause chest pain. But the diagnosis of MI is straightforward for most patients. When the clinical history is typical and there are clear-cut changes on the ECG, start thrombolytic drugs before getting the chest X-ray.

A single laboratory request form or single computerized laboratory panel for patients with chest pain is especially useful. We found that our nurses and emergency department technicians were wasting important time filling out multiple laboratory request forms or ordering multiple tests with the computer. Because it "had to be done" the clerical task assumed its own importance and invariably delayed thrombolytic therapy. Our new "Cardiac Laboratory Panel" includes routine admission laboratories, cardiac enzymes, platelet count, prothrombin time, and activated partial thromboplastin time. *Do not wait* for the laboratory results. If the patient is early in the course of acute MI cardiac enzymes will not be elevated. The results of clotting studies rarely alter the decision to use thrombolytic drugs. The decision to treat is based solely on the ECG and clinical history.

Avoid "routine" arterial blood gases. This may be the third or fourth time we have mentioned this, but it is important to remember. Arterial sticks are responsible for some of the worst complications of thrombolytic therapy we have encountered. We would consider arterial gases only for patients with incipient respiratory failure, or who have advanced obstructive lung disease with respiratory distress. If the patient has already had blood gases drawn, can he or she be considered for thrombolytic therapy? The danger of acute MI is great enough that we would proceed with thrombolytic therapy for a patient who has had blood gases, but we would pay special attention to the arterial puncture site.

We feel that no more than two i.v. lines should be established before administering thrombolytic therapy. We still encounter emergency departments that require three i.v. lines. Rapid administration of the thrombolytic agent is the most important aspect of the patient's care. Most problems that arise early can be managed with two i.v. lines. Starting additional i.v. lines so that other drugs can be given is fine, but it is not necessary to do this before starting thrombolytic therapy. The newly developed, double–lumen intravenous catheter is especially useful (and provides two lines).

The biggest roadblock to using thrombolytic therapy is timidity. The risk of bleeding complications (Chapter 9) and especially the 0.5–1% risk of intracranial bleeding are frightening. *But this is no time to be timid*. While there are risks, the survival and functional benefits of thrombolytic therapy are well established. In the absence of contraindications, the greatest opportunity for your patients with acute Q wave MI lies with thrombolytic therapy. We reiterate that the correct medical motto should not be *premum non nocere*; you will at times unavoidably injure patients with virtually any therapy. Rather, follow the rule that you presently use for all other medical therapies: *play the best odds*.

How to change the system

There is no way one or two enlightened people (doctors, nurses, or hospital administrators) can make these changes. We know because we have struggled with them for more than 1 year in our hospital. To do this right you must have a consensus of opinion and the support and commitment of the medical, nursing, and administrative staffs. A joint committee comprised of representatives of each of these groups has the best opportunity to change treatment patterns in your emergency department. We found that the emergency department nursing staff was especially effective in identifying problems and solutions. They will be more apt to help improve time to therapy if they are involved at the beginning.

One more committee? This hardly seems a way to promote efficiency in any hospital! But this committee may do some good. In addition to establishing a new protocol for treating patients with chest pain in your hospital, the committee should continue to monitor performance.

Role of the hospital administrator

While this book is written for doctors and nurses caring for patients with acute MI, we have a message for hospital administrators. We found it difficult to shorten time to therapy in the emergency department without help from hospital administration. The changes recommended in Table 10.1 can be facilitated enormously by an administrator who is able to coordinate the nursing staff (all shifts), the medical staff, laboratory, X-ray, ECG, and pharmacy into a coherent unit whose goal is more rapid treatment. There is no one else in the hospital who is able to work as effectively with all of these groups. The hospital administrator on our rapid application committee has turned out to be the member with the greatest influence, the facilitator.

A second role for hospital administration has to do with the broader role of the hospital in the community. For thrombolytic therapy to be effective, patients must recognize symptoms of MI early and seek prompt medical attention. We and others have studied specific public education campaigns aimed at getting patients with chest pain to the emergency department earlier. We have found that it is difficult to immediately change patient behavior patterns, but do have anecdotal experience with patients who were directly influenced to come to hospital early because of public education announcements.

First hour program

Our most ambitious public education campaign was the *first hour* program developed with assistance from the American Heart Association, Illinois affiliate. We borrowed the title from a similar program developed 10 years ago in Los Angeles by Lawrence Herman. The title implies that the patient should seek medical attention within the first hour of the onset of symptoms of a heart attack. The program has two facets: first, an emergency department is "certified" as being capable of treating heart attack. The criteria for certification are quite simple, and most experienced and well managed emergency departments already meet them.

The second aspect of the program is that the local hospital publicizes the fact that its emergency department has been "certified" by the *first hour* program as a heart attack center. The focus of the publicity campaign is the education of the public about the warning signs of MI and the need for rapid evaluation. Samples of the public service advertising materials are provided in Figures 10.1, 10.2 and 10.3, and include materials for local print media, radio, and television. These ads underscore the need for treatment of heart attack within 1 hour of the onset of symptoms.

Most hospitals have a budget for public relations and public education and can institute an education program easily. There is tremendous community support for such programs. The programs enhance the image of the hospital and emergency department as well as provide important public education.

The *first hour* program was introduced into 80 communities in central and southern Illinois in 1986–1988. Most had hospitals with less than 100 beds. We studied the effect of the program in one community by reviewing emergency department records the year before starting *first hour* and then 2 years after (Moses, *et al.*). We specifically wondered whether the emergency department would evaluate more patients with chest pain and whether the patients would come to the emergency department earlier after onset of symptoms. One encouraging finding was that the public education program did not precipitate a stampede of panicked citizens into the emergency department. There was no significant increase in emergency department utilization. Unfortunately, we were unable to document any other change in behavior. The time from onset of symptoms to presentation in the emergency department was not changed on average. We did encounter individual patients who developed chest pain and received prompt medical attention because of the *first hour* program. Often they were young people who had heard or read the public service spots which prompted them to seek medical care when they developed symptoms.

A similar public education program was performed in a larger community, Goteborg, Sweden. The length of the education program and its content were similar to *first hour*. These investigators were able to document a small decrease in average length of symptoms before presenting to the emergency department in patients with chest pain, and they attributed this to the public education program.

Perhaps the most important message from these pilot studies is that changing patient behavior in order to reduce time to

AMERICAN HEART ASSOCIATION – ILLINOIS AFFILIATE
FIRST HOUR PROGRAM
Swiss cheese radio P.S.A.s

10 seconds

_____(hospital name)_____ has implemented the American

Heart Association's new *first hour* program. For more information on *first hour* and heart attack prevention, call

_____(name or phone number of hospital)_____

20 seconds

Some people would rather die of embarrassment than admit they're having a heart attack. And die they might, for the average victim waits over 3 hours before seeking medical help.

Call _____(hospital name)_____ for more information on their

first hour program. Learn the warning signs of a heart attack and be prepared to act fast!

30 seconds

There are times when you should ignore a heart attack victim . . . he or she says, "It's just indigestion" . . . or "it's nerves" . . . Unfortunately, the average heart attack victim waits more than 3 hours before seeking medical help. Preventable sudden death often occurs within the *first hour* of onset of symptoms. Call

_____(hospital name and phone number)_____ to learn more

about their *first hour* program. Learn the warning signs of a heart attack and be ready to act fast!

Instructions

Retype the PSAs on your hospital letterhead, filling in the appropriate blank spaces, and forward to your local radio stations. Always provide stations with the name and phone number of the appropriate contact person in your hospital (i.e., Public Relations Director, Hospital Administrator, or person submitting the release).

Fig. 10.1 An example of advertising material used by the *first hour* program in central Illinois and by our hospital's Chest Pain Center. (From the American Heart Association, Illinois Affiliate and St John's Hospital.)

First hour

Swiss cheese news release

For more information contact

_____ (name/phone) _____

For immediate release

(or, for release _____ (date) _____)

(hospital name) joins *first hour* program

_____ (hospital name) _____ has just been given a 2 year

certification from the American Heart Association, Illinois affiliate, as a participant in their new *first hour* program.

The term "first hour" refers to the fact that preventable sudden death often occurs within the first hour of onset of symptoms. Unfortunately, the average heart attack victim waits nearly 3 hours before seeking medical help.

As a participant of the *first hour* program,

_____ (hospital name) _____ meets the Emergency Heart Care

standards developed by the Heart Association for this program. These standards include assurance that appropriate equipment and cardiac drugs are immediately available in the Emergency Room. All personnel in the hospital's Emergency Room must have specific training in emergency cardiac care (also known as Advanced Cardiac Life Support).

By joining the *first hour* program,

_____ (hospital name) _____ has made the committment to

carry on community education campaigns to emphasize the need to recognize warning signs of heart attack and to seek immediate help through the nearest medical facility. Even though

_____ (hospital name) _____ has been recognized for its

standards of emergency cardiac care, the patient and patient's family can sometimes reduce the severity of a heart attack by seeking medical treatment during the first few minutes . . . before major damage occurs to the heart muscle.

_____ (administrator's name) _____ says, "For years, our hospital has

been known for high quality patient care. Participation in the *first hour* program is just another way for

_____ (hospital name) _____ to demonstrate this care."

Fig. 10.2 An example of advertising material used by the *first hour* program in central Illinois and by our hospital's Chest Pain Center. (From the American Heart Association, Illinois Affiliate and St John's Hospital.)

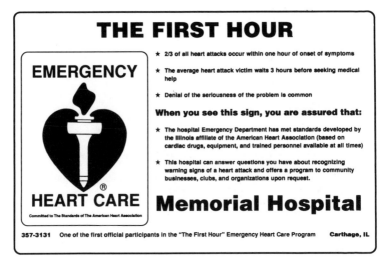

Fig. 10.3 An example of advertising material used by the *first hour* program in central Illinois and by our hospital's Chest Pain Center. (From the American Heart Association, Illinois Affiliate and St John's Hospital.)

presentation to the emergency department requires more than a *brief* community education program. There is no quick fix. Public education requires a long-term commitment, and we see the community hospital as the logical provider of this. In Illinois, the American Heart Association was a willing and suitable collaborator for this program.

A similar approach is to promote the hospital's emergency department as a "Chest Pain Center" (Fig. 10.4). The community education program should encourage patients to come directly to the emergency department with chest pain rather than to their doctor's office. Our medical staff had no difficulty in endorsing this approach. At a time when there is unseemly competition for "market share," public education remains a suitable role for hospitals. It is a "win–win" situation that enhances the image of the hospital and helps patients.

Apart from broad public education, the individual physician should specifically educate high risk patients about the need to seek immediate medical attention in the emergency department if they have symptoms of MI. All of these programs should emphasize that the risk of death and disability can be reduced if the patient heeds early warning signs.

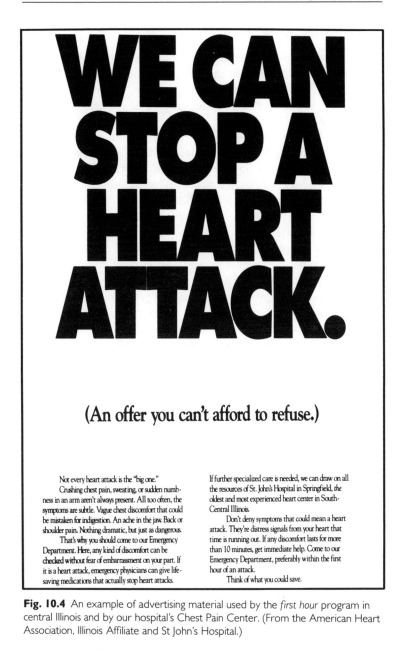

Fig. 10.4 An example of advertising material used by the *first hour* program in central Illinois and by our hospital's Chest Pain Center. (From the American Heart Association, Illinois Affiliate and St John's Hospital.)

Prehospital therapy

There have been studies indicating that administration of thrombolytic agents is feasible in the field or in the ambulance prior to hospital or emergency department admission. The most successful prehospital treatment studies actually sent physicians with the ambulance.

It seems to us unlikely that prehospital therapy will become widespread. It would require a highly skilled emergency medical technician team attending patients with chest pain in the field. Frankly, experienced physicians are often confused about whether thrombolytic therapy is appropriate for a particular patient. Having emergency medical technicians make the decision to treat with thrombolytic agents in cooperation with the emergency department physician may require a level of team work and skill that cannot be practically achieved in most communities. In rural Illinois the ambulance ride to the emergency department is usually short. The greatest impetus for prehospital treatment is the astonishing delay that takes place once the patient reaches the emergency department. With the improvement in response time that we have accomplished in our emergency department, we feel less need for prehospital treatment.

Prehospital treatment would require transmission of the 12-lead ECG to the emergency department. Apart from out of hospital treatment with thrombolytic agents, an ability to transmit a 12-lead ECG from the field has other advantages. A major impediment to early therapy is the delay in obtaining an ECG when the patient reaches the emergency department. Obtaining the 12-lead ECG before the patient's arrival would alert the emergency department staff to the diagnosis and could dramatically shorten time to therapy.

The technology for obtaining and transmitting a 12-lead ECG from the field by the ambulance team is evolving. There are three possibilities. The first uses existing telephone lines. Difficulties with this approach include portability and accessibility of a telephone jack (which many older homes do not have).

A second possibility is radio telemetry. Currently the Federal Communication Commission (FCC) allows ambulances to transmit at 400–500 MHz. There is considerable interference at this frequency prohibiting transmission of a technically adequate 12-lead ECG. Systems are being developed that use 800 MHz transmission, but are not currently approved by the FCC. Radio transmission is also limited by distance. With our current radio telemetry system we are able to to transmit reliably over a distance of 12–15 miles. Long distance transmission is impossible. Direct line transmission of radio signals is blocked by hills, and artifact is easily introduced by atmospheric conditions or other electrical signals.

The third and apparently best technique for transmitting a 12-lead ECG involves the cellular telephone. The quality of the transmitted ECG is excellent. The only limitation is coverage by the cellular network. In rural, central Illinois there are a few areas that cannot be reached by cellular telephone.

A number of companies are working to develop a 12-lead ECG transmission system which would be suitable for ambulance use. One commercially available unit allows transmission of a 12-lead ECG over cellular telephone, instant computer analysis of the ECG, and continuous ECG telemetry using radio transmission at 400 MHz. It also functions as a defibrillator and as an external cardiac pacemaker. The present cost of the unit is approximately $12 000, about 30% more expensive than the standard telemetry–defibrillator unit that is carried by most ambulances.

Selected reading

Aufderheide TP, Hendley GE, Thakur RK, et al. The diagnostic impact of prehospital 12-lead electrocardiography. Annals Emerg Med 1990; 19:1280–87.

GISSI-1. Effectiveness of thrombolytic treatment in acute myocardial infarction. Lancet 1986;1:397–402.

ISIS-2 Collaborative Group. Randomized trial of intravenous strepto-kinase, oral aspirin, both, or neither among 17 187 cases of suspected acute myocardial infarction: ISIS-2*. J Am Coll Cardiol 1988;12: 3–13A.

Karagounis L, Ipsen SK, Jessop MR, et al. Impact of field-transmitted electrocardiography on time to in-hospital thrombolytic therapy in acute myocardial infarction. Am J Cardiol 1990;66:786–91.

Kereiakes DJ, Weaver WD, Anderson JL, et al. Time delays in the diagnosis and treatment of acute myocardial infarction: a tale of eight cities. Report from the Prehospital Study Group and the Cincinnati Heart Project. Am Heart J 1990;120:773–79.

Moses HW, Bartolozzi JJ, Koester DL, et al. Reducing delay in the emergency room in administration of thrombolytic therapy for myocardial infarction associated with ST elevation. Am J Cardiol 1991;68:251–53.

Moses HW, Engelking N, Taylor GJ, et al. Effect of a two-year public education campaign on reducing response time of patients with symptoms of acute myocardial infarction. Am J Cardiol 1991;68:249–51.

Chapter 11
Late prognosis after MI and long-term therapy

Prognosis after MI

Prognosis without thrombolytic therapy

Natural history studies of coronary artery disease following MI in the prethrombolytic therapy era indicate a 5-year mortality rate of 40–50% (Fig. 7.2). Patients with large MI and LVEF <40% had much worse prognosis than those with smaller acute MI (Table 1.3). With later, 5-year follow-up, *multivessel coronary disease* also predicted recurrent ischemia and mortality. By 5 years there had been progression of disease, and many patients returned with another round of ischemic events.

Complex ventricular ectopy on a Holter monitor just before hospital discharge also predicts high mortality during the year after acute MI. However, studies incorporating multivariate statistical analysis discovered that complex ectopy is not an independent predictor of mortality. Instead, it is closely tied to low LVEF. Patients with LV failure have complex ectopy, and vice versa. Sudden cardiac death is common in postinfarction patients, especially those with LV depression.

When these data linking increased mortality to ventricular arrhythmias became available, it appeared reasonable to treat high risk patients with antiarrhythmic drugs. The CAST study was the first randomized trial of antiarrhythmic drug therapy after acute MI. It compared encainide or flecainide therapy with placebo in postinfarction patients who had complex ventricular ectopy on a 24-hour Holter monitor. The result was surprising: patients on antiarrhythmic therapy had increased mortality at 10 months (Fig. 11.1). The proarrhythmic effects of these drugs apparently outweighed any beneficial actions, and patients treated with either flecainide and encainide had a higher risk of sudden death. Because of this study our approach to antiarrhythmic therapy after MI has been drastically altered. Drug therapy is

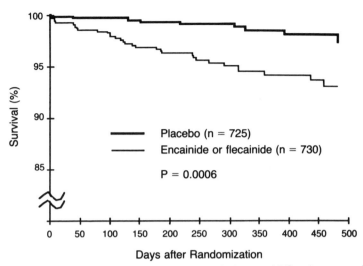

Fig. 11.1 The CAST study result describing survival among 1445 patients treated with encainide or flecainide, or placebo. Cardiac arrest or arrhythmia was the cause of death. (From Rogers, *et al. N Engl J Med* 1989;321:406.)

reserved for those with symptomatic or sustained VT or VF, and therapy is often guided by electrophysiologic testing. The CAST study is ongoing. Ethmozine did not have the proarrhythmic potential of flecainide or encainide and is still being studied.

Non-Q wave infarction merits special mention. These are "small" heart attacks; peak CK is lower, and predischarge LVEF is higher than with Q wave MI. It was initially assumed that patients with non-Q wave MI have a good prognosis. However, when these patients were followed prospectively after MI they were found to have a high rate of recurrent infarction. Their 1 year mortality rate was similar to that of patients admitted to hospital with Q wave MI. From these studies we have learned that non-Q wave infarction is an unstable coronary syndrome. These patients often have tight and ragged stenosis involving a major coronary branch, but incomplete injury. Non-Q wave infarction is considered an indication for angiography and possible revascularization.

Prognosis after thrombolytic therapy

A blanket statement cannot be made about prognosis for all patients after thrombolytic therapy. Successful thrombolysis (an open infarct artery at catheterization) conveys a survival benefit. But subsequent therapy also influences prognosis. Our clinical experience and our assessment of the published experience of others suggests that patients who have early revascularization will be more stable during follow-up.

Using our treatment strategy of thrombolytic therapy applied early in the course of MI, anticoagulant therapy including heparin and aspirin, then early angiography and possibly revascularization, we have consistently observed 5–7% in-hospital mortality. A series of 180 survivors of hospitalization after Q wave MI treated before 1983 has been the subject of two follow-up studies, at 20 months and again at 6 years. The 6-year mortality rate in the 180 survivors was 12%, suggesting much better long-term survival with this treatment approach when compared with traditional, prethrombolytic therapy management. It is noteworthy that all the patients in our study had ST segment elevation, or Q wave MI. None had non-Q wave infarction. Both the 20-month and 6-year follow-up studies found that an open infarct artery at catheterization was an important predictor of survival (Fig. 1.1). In fact, multivariate analysis confirmed that an open infarct artery at catheterization within 24 hours was an independent predictor of 6 year survival, and LVEF was not.

What is responsible for this excellent long-term survival? Is it thrombolytic therapy and salvage of myocardium? Or is good long-term survival a product of revascularization? Patients with an open infarct artery more commonly had a revascularization procedure. It is difficult to be sure, but using multivariate statistical analysis, an open infarct artery at catheterization ("successful thrombolysis") was an independent predictor of survival, and coronary artery revascularization was not. Nevertheless, we suspect that protecting the open artery is critical in preserving the benefits of early reperfusion. We attribute the late survival result to a treatment strategy including both thrombolytic therapy and early revascularization.

Others have suggested that late benefits of thrombolytic therapy cannot be assessed in studies where a high percentage of patients have revascularization. We take almost the opposite viewpoint: the infarct artery is unstable after thrombolysis and is prone to reocclusion with loss of the benefits of reperfusion. We consider it unlikely that the maximum benefit of early reperfusion can be assessed without early revascularization (Chapter 7).

There are no late follow-up studies of patients who received

Table 11.1 Infarct artery morphology: 39 patients with <50% stenosis (From Taylor, *et al.*, 1991)

	Normal-appearing artery	Minimal stenosis: ragged plaque surface	Minimal stenosis: smooth plaque surface
Prevalence	8/39	17/39	13/39
Mechanisms of occlusion	Spasm, thrombosis, and plaque	Thrombosis, plaque, and spasm	Thrombosis, plaque, and spasm
Reinfarction (51 ± 12 month follow-up)	1/8	0/17	4/13

thrombolytic therapy and were then treated medically, without revascularization. The TIMI-2A trial described 1-year follow-up. Patients in the "conservative strategy group" of the study, who did not have early angiography unless they had a positive exercise-RNA or symptoms, had a 39% rate of revascularization at 1 year. This high rate of revascularization contradicts the popular interpretation of the TIMI-2 study that patients can be treated medically (or ignored) after thrombolytic therapy and will do well. On the contrary, patients in the conservative wing of the TIMI-2A study had their share of problems and needed careful follow-up.

Patients with "minimal" coronary disease

Coronary thrombosis and occlusion usually develop in arteries that are tightly stenosed. In a series of 580 patients having thrombolytic therapy and angiography within 3 days, we found 39 (7%) who had <50% stenosis of the infarct artery (Taylor, *et al.*, 1991).

The pathophysiology of acute coronary occlusion probably involves the interaction of atherosclerotic plaque, thrombosis, and arterial spasm. The angiographic appearance of these "minimally diseased" infarct arteries may provide insight into the mechanisms of occlusion (Table 11.1). One group of patients had normal appearing arteries with no irregularity at all. We assume that coronary artery spasm may have played a prominent role in development of MI in these patients. There are clinical data implicating spasm in some of them. One required intracoronary nitroglycerin therapy to maintain an open infarct artery after initial thrombolysis with intracoronary STK (Moses, *et al.*, 1983). Another of these patients was asymptomatic after his anterior MI on high dose nifedipine therapy. While on a business trip he ran out of medicine, and had recurrent anterior MI 18 hours after taking the last pill.

A majority of the patients with minimal disease had luminal irregularity, presumably atherosclerotic plaque. These patients fell into two categories (Table 11.1). One group had ragged plaque surface with scalloping, haziness of the plaque margin, or persistent thrombus (appearing as a filling defect on the angiogram). This ragged plaque surface suggests thrombus formation as a dominant mechanism of arterial occlusion for these patients. Similar morphologic studies of patients with angina pectoris indicate that smooth plaque surface is most common in patients with chronic stable angina. Those with unstable angina more likely have ragged plaque surface.

A third group of patients with minimal coronary artery narrowing had smooth plaque surface (Table 11.1). In their case, the relative contribution of spasm and thrombosis to the pathophysiology of infarction is uncertain.

The patients with minimal disease were treated medically; revascularization was recommended for just two of them who had multivessel coronary disease. Medical therapy included aspirin and calcium channel blockers for all patients. Those who had ragged plaque and any suggestion of active thrombus also were treated with warfarin for 2–3 months in addition to aspirin. The minimal disease patients were followed 51 ± 12 months. Despite aggressive medical therapy 5 (13%) had recurrent MI, 1 week to 36 months after the initial infarction. By contrast, we reported just 3% recurrent MI in our initial series of 180 patients during 20-month follow-up after thrombolytic therapy. Most patients in this series had critical coronary stenosis and 61% had revascularization (Sutton, *et al.*, 1986). Minimal stenosis does not mean minimal risk after MI and thrombolysis.

Long-term therapy after thrombolysis

Late therapy is largely dictated by the treatment strategy after reperfusion. Patients who have had coronary artery bypass surgery following thrombolytic therapy for MI are managed like patients who have had bypass surgery for other coronary syndromes. They are treated indefinitely with aspirin. Prophylactic antianginal therapy is not indicated.

Patients who have had angioplasty are also treated with aspirin. We treat these patients at the time of angioplasty with calcium channel blockers and send them home on calcium antagonists for 3–6 months. This is common practice, but it is an approach that has not been validated by randomized trials. Should these patients be on beta blocker therapy? Again, the issue has not been studied, but we have not used beta blocker therapy prophylactically after PTCA. Restenosis has been described in 20–35% of patients after PTCA. No study has indicated that the process of restenosis is any different for patients having angioplasty after thrombolytic therapy than it is for patients having PTCA for angina pectoris.

Patients managed medically following thrombolytic therapy, who have not had angiography, probably should have aggressive, prophylactic antianginal therapy. This seems especially important in light of the high risk of silent ischemia (Chapter 7). There has been no systematic study of these asymptomatic patients indicating a correct approach; no trials have compared antianginal drugs with placebo.

A number of drug classes should be considered for use after MI in thrombolytic therapy:

Beta adrenergic blocking drugs

Large studies from the prethrombolytic therapy era have shown that beta adrenergic blockers reduce late postinfarction mortality by 25%. These trials excluded patients with CHF. As a result, late mortality in these studies was low for both placebo and drug treatment groups. Beta blocker therapy reduced the incidence of recurrent ischemia. Less sudden death suggested an antiarrhythmic action as well.

A TIMI-2 substudy evaluated metoprolol for patients after thrombolytic therapy. One group of patients was treated with metoprolol early in the course of treatment, within 2 hours of starting rt-PA. The second group had oral therapy begun on day 6 after MI. The primary endpoints were LV function and survival. Predischarge ejection fraction was identical for the two groups as was hospital mortality. But patients who had immediate, intravenous therapy had a lower incidence of reinfarction and recurrent chest pain at day 6 (the time to therapy was begun in the "delayed" treatment group).

The effect of chronic beta blocker therapy on late survival after acute MI and thrombolytic therapy has not been studied. But we would recommend prophylactic beta blockade for patients following a conservative, medical treatment strategy.

Calcium antagonists

There have been no studies of calcium antagonist therapy after thrombolytic therapy. The diltiazem reinfarction trials found less reinfarction during the 2 weeks after acute, non-Q wave MI. We have suggested that patients after thrombolytic therapy may be similar to those with non-Q wave MI: both have incomplete injury and an unstable coronary lesion. Theoretically, calcium antagonist therapy would block spasm and protect patients following thrombolysis. Within our practice group we have differing opinions; some recommend combined therapy with calcium antagonists and beta blockers in addition to aspirin as "maximal medical therapy" for asymptomatic patients managed medically after thrombolysis. Others among us consider aspirin plus beta blockers adequate prophylaxis.

We would caution you to remember the possibility of silent ischemia and silent ischemic injury in patients after thrombolytic therapy and MI (Chapter 7). Calcium blocker therapy has proven useful for patients with known coronary artery disease, intermittent angina pectoris, but also silent ischemia. A change in general condition or exercise tolerance, or the appearance of new arrhythmias should prompt a search for recurrent ischemia.

Antiplatelet therapy

We recommend that all patients who have had thrombolytic therapy for MI, including those who have had revascularization procedures, be on antiplatelet therapy. We currently treat patients with 1 enteric coated aspirin daily. Again, this treatment approach has not been validated by randomized trials. There is enough background literature on the benefits of low dose aspirin for patients with atherosclerotic vascular disease that most would consider this recommendation noncontroversial and not worthy of a large and expensive clinical trial.

Warfarin

Anticoagulation with warfarin may be useful in two different settings. We have mentioned patients with noncritical (<50%)

infarct artery stenosis with ragged and ulcerated plaque surface. We have commonly treated these patients with aspirin plus warfarin for 2–3 months after thrombolytic therapy, and with aspirin alone thereafter. There is an increased risk of GI bleeding on this combination. Careful monitoring of therapy is essential, and antacid therapy may be considered as well.

A second indication for warfarin anticoagulation is LV mural thrombus. This is most common in patients with large anterior infarction. The risk of mural thrombus is reduced but not eliminated by thrombolytic therapy. Peripheral embolization may be prevented in these patients by warfarin therapy. We routinely get screening echocardiograms in patients with anterior MI prior to hospital discharge, and anticoagulate those with mural thrombus. The proper duration of therapy is uncertain. If the anterior and apical LV segments are akinetic, thrombus may reform when warfarin is discontinued. Serial echocardiograms would be important after stopping anticoagulants. Patients who have had an embolic event probably should have indefinite anticoagulation.

Long acting nitrates

We do not currently recommend prophylactic, long acting nitroglycerin therapy for asymptomatic patients after MI, regardless of whether or not they have had thrombolytic therapy.

ACE inhibitors

Patients who have LV dysfunction (ejection fraction <40–45%) after MI may benefit from ACE inhibitors. Two studies have found that long-term captopril therapy improves LV geometry and systolic function. Pfeffer, et al., studied patients with anterior infarction. Sharpe and colleagues found similar benefits in patients with inferior MI. There have been no studies testing the effect of afterload reduction therapy on late survival after MI. But randomized trials of captopril and enalapril have found improved survival in patients with CHF, and these trials included patients with ischemic cardiomyopathy.

None of these studies were performed in patients after thrombolytic therapy. Nevertheless, we currently recommend afterload reduction therapy using ACE inhibitors in patients who have had thrombolytic therapy and who have LVEF <40%.

Progression of coronary artery disease

In my 12th year in practice I find that one-fourth of the patients I take to the catheterization laboratory have been there with me before. Coronary artery disease is progressive, and it is common for patients to return in 4–8 year cycles with progression of disease. While the developments of the last decade including thrombolytic therapy and interventional cardiology have been impressive, we will not be able to offer our patients a "cure" until we are able to halt progression of atherosclerosis.

We may be close to that. Recently Brown, *et al.*, described a serial angiographic study of patients with moderate hyperlipidemia who were treated with either colestipol (the "control group"), colestipol + niacin, or colestipol + lovastatin. The aggressive lipid altering regimen blocked progression of disease in 75–80% of patients. Even more impressive was the observation that 39% of patients treated with niacin + colestipol and 32% treated with lovastatin + colestipol had regression of atherosclerotic plaque (Table 11.2).

Brown's study may be a glimpse into the future. We may be approaching a time when progression of disease can be reliably stopped for most patients. The 1980s was the decade of interventional cardiology including thrombolytic therapy. The 1990s may be remembered as the decade of metabolic control of atherosclerosis.

It is noteworthy that the patients in Brown's study who followed a rigid, low cholesterol diet had the best results. Aggressive risk factor modification programs aimed at cigarette smoking, diabetes, hypertension, diet, and exercise all remain important.

Long-term follow-up

Studies that have examined the value of serial stress testing and even serial angiography have found that neither technique allows reliable prediction of the future. More specifically, a yearly stress ECG cannot be trusted to identify the patient who is destined to develop new symptoms or have recurrent MI. Similarly, serial angiography studies have found that predicting the site of disease progression is impossible. The borderline lesion observed in an artery may not be the one that progresses and causes future symptoms. For example, a patient with a borderline stenosis in the right coronary artery on an initial angiogram may well

Table 11.2 Intensive lipid-lowering therapy: a serial angiographic study (From Brown, et al. 146 male patients with elevated apolipoprotein B, coronary artery disease at initial catheterization, and follow-up catheterization 2 and a half years later)

Drug regimen*	LDL (%)	HDL (%)	Progression of plaque (%)	Regression of plaque (%)
Colestipol	− 7	+ 5	46	11
Lovastatin + colestipol	−46	+15	21	32
Niacin + colestipol	−32	+43	25	39

* Lovastatin 20 mg twice a day, niacin 1 g four times a day, colestipol 10 g three times a day.

develop ischemic symptoms because of progression of disease in another vessel. It is for these reasons that we seldom advise "routine" follow-up angiography or even stress tests for asymptomatic patients who have had coronary artery bypass graft surgery.

Patients who have had angioplasty may be a special case. There is a 25% chance for restenosis of the dilated artery, usually within 6 months of the procedure. A stress ECG 6 months following PTCA is a reliable screening test for restenosis. This may be especially helpful for patients who have had angioplasty following thrombolytic therapy, as silent ischemia may be more common.

For the same reason follow-up stress testing for patients who are treated "conservatively" after thrombolytic therapy also may be useful. Exercise studies and especially exercise studies which include assessment of myocardial perfusion (an exercise tallium scan), or LV function (exercise echocardiogram or RNA) may help detect silent ischemia. In similar fashion, we have recommended follow-up angiography for a minority of patients having thrombolytic therapy who have especially unstable appearing coronary artery plaque and who are being treated medically.

Selected reading

Brown G, Albers JJ, Fisher LD, *et al*. Regression of coronary artery disease as a result of intensive lipid-lowering therapy in men with high levels of apolipoprotein B. N Engl J Med 1990;323:1289–98.

Kannel WB, Sorlie P, McNamara PM. Prognosis after initial myocardial infarction: The Framingham Study. Am J Cardiol 1979;44:53–9.

Moses HW, Taylor GJ, Asali Z, Brewer TE. Coronary artery spasm causing myocardial infarction. IMJ 1983;163:265–68.

Pfeffer MA, Lamas GA, Vaughan DE, Parisi AF, Braunwald E. Effect of captopril on progressive ventricular dilatation after anterior myocardial infarction. N Engl J Med 1988;319:80–6.

Roberts, R, Rogers WJ, Mueller HS, et al. Immediate versus deferred B-Blockade following thrombolytic therapy in patients with acute myocardial infarction. Results of the thrombolysis in myocardial infarction (TIMI) II-B Study. Circulation 1991;83:422–37.

Rogers WJ, Epstein AE, Arciniegas JG, et al. Special Report. Preliminary report: Effect of encainide and flecainide on mortality in a randomized trial of arrhythmia suppression after myocardial infarction. N Engl J Med 1989;321:406–12.

Sharpe N, Smith H, Murphy J, Hannan S. Treatment of patients with symptomless left ventricular dysfunction after myocardial infarction. Lancet 1988;1:255–59.

Sutton JM, Taylor GJ, Mikell FL, et al. Thrombolytic therapy followed by early revascularization for acute myocardial infarction. Am J Cardiol 1986;57:1227–31.

Taylor GJ, Mikell FL, Koester DL, et al. Infarct artery and lesion morphology in patients with minimal stenosis after thrombolytic therapy for acute MI. JACC 1991;17:246A (abstr).

Taylor GJ, Moses HW, Korsmeyer C, et al. Six-year survival after coronary thrombolysis and early revascularization (Unpublished data).

TIMI Study Group. Comparison of invasive and conservative strategies after treatment with intravenous tissue plasminogen activator in acute myocardial infarction. N Engl J Med 1989;320:618–27.

Yusuf S, Peto R, Lewis J, Collins R, Sleight P. Beta blockade during and after myocardial infarction: An overview of the randomized trials. Prog Cardiovasc Dis 1985;27:335–71.

Yusuf S, Sleight P, Held P, McMahon S. Routine medical management of acute myocardial infarction. Lessons from overviews of recent randomized controlled trials. Circulation 1990;82(Suppl II):17–134.

Appendix 1
Annotated references: a survey of randomized trials

Appendix 1 will catalog and provide brief reviews of selected trials of thrombolytic therapy.

Trials comparing thrombolytic therapy with placebo (Tables 1.1, 1.2)

Mortality trials

1 GISSI-1 (First study of the Gruppo Italiano per lo studio della streptochinasi nell'infarto miocardico). Effectiveness of intravenous thrombolytic treatment in acute myocardial infarction. Lancet 1986;1:397–402.

This was the first large randomized trial which proved that thrombolytic therapy improves survival. It was an unblinded study of 11 806 patients who were treated with intravenous STK or placebo. Mortality was 10.7% with STK vs 13% for controls. The beneficial effect was related to the time to treatment; those treated within 1 hour of the onset of MI had the greatest benefit, a 47% reduction in mortality. This study found no significant improvement in survival in patients older than 65 years, but did indicate a favorable trend. Adjunctive therapy was not controlled by the study, and a minority of patients were treated with either heparin or aspirin. The survival benefit of intravenous STK was maintained at 1 year follow-up. During follow-up, symptomatic reinfarction was twice as common in the STK group. This is the expected result, as patients who have had thrombolytic therapy and have an open infarct artery are at risk for reocclusion.

2 ISIS-2 (Second International Study of Infarct Survival) Collaborative Group. Randomised trial of intravenous streptokinase, oral aspirin, both, or neither among 17 187 cases of suspected acute myocardial infarction: ISIS-2. Lancet 1988;2:349–60.

ISIS-1 was a study of beta blocker therapy, not thrombolytic therapy. The ISIS-2 trial randomly treated 17 187 patients with STK, placebo, aspirin, or STK + aspirin. Both STK and aspirin alone produced a reduction in 5-week mortality. The combination of STK and aspirin was better than either agent alone (Fig. 8.4). Aspirin therapy also reduced nonfatal reinfarction and nonfatal stroke. ISIS-2 also found that patients treated earliest had best results. But it also reported that patients treated as late as 13–24 hours after onset of pain had reduced mortality with thrombolytic therapy. Heparin was not used in this study. Patients with BBB and elderly patients benefited from thrombolytic therapy. Patients with ST segment depression had no significant benefit.

3 ASSET (Anglo-Scandinavian study of early thrombolysis). Wilcox RG, von der Lippe G, Olsson CG, *et al*. Trial of tissue plasminogen activator for mortality reduction in acute myocardial infarction. Lancet 1988;2:525–30.

This randomized trial compared rt-PA plus heparin with placebo plus heparin (5011 patients with chest pain <5 hours). Thrombolytic therapy clearly improved survival (Table 1.2). The entry criterion was "clinical suspicion of MI"; 72% of patients had "definite, probable or possible" MI, and the remainder did not. Those with an abnormal ECG on admission benefited most from rt-PA therapy. There were more hemorrhagic strokes in the rt-PA group (0.3% vs 0.08% with placebo), but there was no difference in the total incidence of stroke at 1 month when comparing rt-PA and placebo therapy.

4 Kennedy JW, Martin GV, Davis KB, *et al*. The Western Washington intravenous streptokinase in acute myocardial infarction randomized trial. Circulation 1988;77:345–52.

This was a randomized, unblinded trial of intravenous STK or standard therapy in 368 patients. Mean time to treatment was 3.5 hours. At 14 days mortality in the STK group was 6.3% compared with 9.6% in the control group ($p = 0.23$). A significant reduction in mortality was noted in patients with anterior MI. Patients treated in <3 hours tended to have lower mortality. The survival benefit in patients with anterior infarction was maintained at 2-year follow-up.

5 AIMS (APSAC Intervention Mortality Study). AIMS Trial Study Group. Effect of intravenous APSAC on mortality after acute myocardial infarction: Preliminary report of a placebo-controlled clinical trial. Lancet 1990;335:427–31.

This was a randomized, trial comparing APSAC with placebo. The endpoint was 30-day mortality. The 1258 patients were treated within 6 hours of onset of MI. APSAC reduced 30-day mortality by 50% (Table 1.2). All patients received intravenous heparin, then warfarin for 3 months. Those without contraindication were discharged on beta blockade. A survival benefit was observed in elderly as well as young patients.

LV function and infarct artery patency trials

6 ISAM (Intravenous streptokinase in acute myocardial infarction). ISAM Study Group. A prospective trial of intravenous streptokinase in acute myocardial infarction (ISAM): Mortality, morbidity and infarct size at 21 days. N Engl J Med 1986;314: 1465–71.

This study of 1741 patients treated randomly with intravenous STK or placebo had LV function and infarct size as endpoints. Time to peak CK was shorter, and the area under the CK-MB curve was smaller in the STK group. A majority of the patients had angiography 3–4 weeks after MI, and patients treated with STK had higher global and regional ejection fraction. The rate of intracranial bleeding was 0.5% in the STK group. STK caused no increase in VF.

7 White HD, Norris RM, Brown MA, *et al*. Effect of intravenous streptokinase on left ventricular function and early survival after acute myocardial infarction. N Engl J Med 1987;317:850–55.

This was a double-blind trial of STK vs placebo in 219 patients with first MI randomized within 4 hours of onset of chest pain. Those without contraindications were also treated with intravenous propranolol early during infarction. Heparin was given for 2 days, and patients were treated with aspirin + dipyridamole until cardiac catheterization at 3 weeks. LVEF was 6 percentage points higher with STK (59% vs 53%). Benefits were noted in patients with both anterior and inferior infarction. LVEF was improved regardless of whether propranolol was given.

8 Guerci AD, Gerstenblith G, Brinker JA, *et al*. A randomized trial of intravenous tissue plasminogen activator for acute myocardial infarction with subsequent randomization to elective coronary angioplasty. N Engl J Med 1987;317:1613–18.

Patients presenting within 4 hours of onset of MI were randomly treated with rt-PA or placebo. Patients receiving rt-PA had global LVEF that was 6 percentage points higher.

Eighty-five of these patients were randomly assigned to receive angioplasty or no angioplasty on the third hospital day. Angioplasty did not influence predischarge ejection fraction at rest. But it did improve the response of ejection fraction to exercise and it reduced the incidence of postinfarction angina.

9 TPAT (Tissue plasminogen activator trial). Morgan CD, Roberts RS, Haq A, *et al*. Coronary patency, infarct size and left ventricular function after thrombolytic therapy for acute myocardial infarction: Results from the tissue plasminogen activator: Toronto (TPAT) placebo-controlled trial. J Am Coll Cardiol 1991;17:1451–57.

This was a randomized trial in 108 patients treated with rt-PA or placebo. Infarct artery patency was the primary endpoint. But a more interesting endpoint was LV function. Radionuclide angiograms were done early and again on day 9 after treatment. Infarct zone ejection fraction improved by 10 percentage points between early and late studies when the infarct artery was open and by only 5 percentage points if it was occluded ($p = 0.05$).

10 National Heart Foundation of Australia Coronary Thrombolysis Group. Coronary thrombolysis and myocardial salvage by tissue plasminogen activator given up to 4 hours after onset of myocardial infarction. Lancet 1988;1:203–08.

This was a small study of 144 patients randomized within 4 hours of onset of MI to rt-PA or placebo. All patients also received intravenous heparin. LVEF was 6 percentage points higher for the rt-PA treated patients 1 week postinfarction, with greatest benefit observed in patients with anterior infarction.

11 Verstraete M, Brower RW, Collen D, *et al*. Double-blind randomised trial of intravenous tissue-type plasminogen activator versus placebo in acute myocardial infarction. Lancet 1985;2: 965–69.

This was a double-blind, randomized trial of 129 patients with first MI treated with rt-PA or placebo. The endpoint was infarct artery patency 90 minutes after starting thrombolytic therapy. The infarct artery was patent in 61% of patients treated with rt-PA vs 21% with placebo. Two hours after starting rt-PA, circulating fibrinogen level had fallen to 52% of the starting value.

12 The Thrombolysis Early in Acute Heart Attack Trial Study Group. Very early thrombolytic therapy in suspected acute myocardial infarction. Am J Cardiol 1990;65:401–07.

This was a placebo-controlled trial of 352 patients comparing rt-PA and placebo. It included patients who were evaluated within 165 minutes of onset of MI. No ECG criteria were required, and 152 patients did not have ST segment elevation at entry (79% of these did not prove to have MI). Endpoints were infarct size, LV function, and exercise capacity at 30 days. Patients treated with rt-PA had increased LVEF and a significantly decreased enzymatic infarct size. There was no benefit in the subgroup without ST segment elevation on the initial ECG. Only 58 patients developed Q waves in the rt-PA group (vs 82 in the placebo group, $p = 0.01$), and the authors stated that "the infarct pattern is shifted from Q-wave to non Q-wave infarcts by rt-PA."

13 APSIM (Anisoylated plasminogen streptokinase in myocardial infarction). Bassand JP, Machecourt J, Cassagnes J, *et al*. Multicenter trial of APSAC in acute myocardial infarction: Effects on infarct size and left ventricular function. J Am Coll Cardiol 1989; 13: 988–97.

This was a randomized, unblinded trial comparing APSAC with conventional heparin therapy. The APSAC group had heparin started 4 hours after initial treatment. Coronary angiography was performed 4 days later and patients had RNA predischarge. Infarct artery patency was 77% in the APSAC group and 36% in the heparin group on day 4. Predischarge ejection fraction was higher for the APSAC group. Thallium-201 tomography indicated smaller infarction with APSAC.

Randomized trials which compared thrombolytic agents (Table 4.2)

Mortality trials

1 GISSI-2 (Second study of the Gruppo Italiano per lo Studio della Sopravvivenza nell'Infarto Miocardico). A factorial randomised trial of alteplase versus streptokinase and heparin versus no heparin among 12 490 patients with acute myocardial infarction. Lancet 1990;336:65–71.

This was a randomized unblinded trial comparing four treatment combinations: (STK, rt-PA, and each with subcutaneous heparin). In the absence of contraindications, all patients were treated with aspirin and intravenous atenolol. There was no difference in mortality between the two thrombolytic agents (overall mortality 8.8%). Addition of heparin did not improve the mortality rate. Other endpoints included clinical heart failure and ejection fraction ≤35%; these endpoints were also unaffected by treatment assignment. The incidence of hemorrhagic stroke was the same in all treatment groups.

2 The International Study Group. In-hospital mortality and clinical course of 20 891 patients with suspected acute myocardial infarction randomised between alteplase and streptokinase with or without heparin. Lancet 1990;336:71–75.

This random trial included the GISSI-2 patients (12 490) and 8401 patients who were treated elsewhere (a total study population of 20 891 patients). Like GISSI-2, patients were randomized to treatment with rt-PA, STK, or each drug with subcutaneous heparin. This study confirmed no difference in hospital mortality between rt-PA and STK, with or without heparin (overall mortality rate 8.6%). More strokes were reported with rt-PA than STK (1.3% vs 1%), while more major bleeding episodes were reported with STK than rt-PA (0.9% vs 0.6%). The addition of subcutaneous heparin was also associated with more serious bleeding, but did not effect incidence of stroke.

3 ISIS-3 (Third International Study of Infarct Survival). Presented at the annual meeting of the American College of Cardiology, Atlanta, Georgia, March 1991.

This study randomly treated 39 913 patients with rt-PA, STK, or APSAC. The mortality rate was similar among the three drug groups (overall mortality rate 10.5%, Table 4.2). Although the risk of bleeding was similar with each drug study, intracranial bleeding occurred more frequently with rt-PA than STK (0.7% vs 0.5%, Figs. 9.2, 9.3) Patients were also randomly treated with subcutaneous heparin + aspirin or aspirin alone. Heparin did not influence the mortality rates with rt-PA or STK. A small subset was treated with intravenous heparin (physician preference rather than study design), and these patients had a higher incidence of intracranial bleeding. Hypotension was observed in patients in each drug group with the highest incidence in patients treated with APSAC.

4 GUSTO (Global utilization of streptokinase and t-PA for occluded coronary arteries).

This is the newest of the randomized trials and it is still in progress. An estimated 40 000 patients will be randomly treated with rt-PA or STK, and mortality is the primary endpoint. All patients receiving rt-PA will be treated with intravenous heparin. Patients on STK will be randomly allocated to intravenous and subcutaneous heparin groups. All patients will be treated with aspirin and intravenous atenolol. Specific issues that will be addressed by the GUSTO trial include the following: (1) Does an open infarct artery early after thrombolytic therapy predict a survival benefit? (2) Does combination therapy with rt-PA and STK improve survival? (3) Is subcutaneous as good as intravenous heparin in patients treated with STK? (4) Is accelerated dosing of rt-PA with front-loading and a shorter infusion time more effective?

LV function trials

5 White HD, Rivers JT, Maslowski AH, *et al.* Effect of intravenous streptokinase as compared with that of tissue plasminogen activator on left ventricular function after first myocardial infarction. N Engl J Med 1989;320:817–21.

This study from Auckland, New Zealand, randomly assigned 270 patients to rt-PA or STK therapy. Patients were treated on average 2.5 hours after onset of chest pain. All received aspirin, dipyridamole, and intravenous heparin. Beta blocker therapy was started about the third day after MI in the absence of contraindications. Nitrates and calcium blockers were prescribed only for postinfarction angina. Catheterization was performed 3 weeks after MI. Global LVEF and regional LV function were identical in both drug groups. Infarct artery patency rates were also similar (75%). Clinical reinfarction occurred in 5% of patients. See Chapter 4 for a more complete discussion.

6 CITTS (Central Illinois thrombolytic therapy study). Taylor GJ, Moses HW, Becker LC, *et al.* Comparison of intravenous tissue plasminogen activator (rt-PA) and streptokinase therapy for acute ST-segment elevation myocardial infarction: Improved regional wall motion in patients with anterior infarction treated with rt-PA. In press.

This randomized, "observer-blinded" study of 253 patients compared rt-PA and STK therapy. It is identical to the study of White, *et al.*, with one major exception: patients had angiography within 2 days of acute MI and 61% had early revascularization (two-thirds having bypass surgery and one-third having angioplasty). Global LVEF was similar in the two drug groups. However, patients with anterior MI who were treated with rt-PA had slightly better regional contractility than those receiving STK. We consider the results suggestive rather than conclusive, and we feel that this should be interpreted as a pilot study. Perhaps it indicates a need for randomized trials incorporating early revascularization and coronary artery bypass surgery as a part of the treatment strategy (Chapter 4).

Studies of infarct artery patency

7 TIMI-1 (First study of thrombolysis in myocardial infarction). The TIMI Study Group. Special Report. The Phase I findings. N Engl J Med 1985;312:932–36.

Chesebro JH, Knatterud G, Roberts R, *et al.* Thrombolysis in myocardial infarction (TIMI) trial, Phase I: a comparison between intravenous tissue plasminogen activator and intravenous streptokinase. Circulation 1987;76:142–54.

Sheehan FH, Braunwald E, Canner P, *et al.* The effect of intravenous thrombolytic therapy on left ventricular function: a report on tissue-type plasminogen activator and streptokinase from the Thrombolysis in Myocardial Infarction (TIMI Phase I) Trial. Circulation 1987;75:817–29.

Rao A, Pratt C, Berke A, *et al.* Thrombolysis in myocardial infarction (TIMI) trial — Phase I: Hemorrhagic manifestations and changes in plasma fibrinogen and the fibrinolytic system in patients treated with recombinant tissue plasminogen activator and streptokinase. J Am Coll Cardiol 1988;11:1–11.

The TIMI-1 trial is perhaps the most influential study of thrombolytic therapy yet completed. It was the first drug comparison trial. Because of the result, rt-PA has been considered the drug of choice by a large number of physicians in the United States (and certainly by Wall Street). The trial included 290 patients randomly treated with rt-PA or STK. Arterial patency was the primary endpoint. To document occlusion of the infarct artery, therapy was delayed until a pretreatment angiogram was obtained. For this reason intravenous thrombolytic therapy was started late, on average 4.8 hours after onset of MI. Patency after 90 minutes of drug infusion was 62% in patients treated with rt-PA and 31% in patients treated with STK ($p < 0.001$). There was no significant difference in any other clinical endpoint. Follow-up LVEF was similar in the two treatment groups. The astonishing difference in arterial patency has not been confirmed by subsequent trials employing earlier thrombolytic therapy (Table 4.2). TIMI-1 thus underscores the importance of early therapy, suggests that rt-PA may be a "faster" thrombolytic agent than STK, and also indicates that rt-PA is more effective later in the course of infarction when thrombus is more mature.

8 ECSG (European Cooperative Study Group). Verstraete M, Bory M, Collen D, *et al.* Randomised trial of intravenous recombinant tissue-type plasminogen activator versus intravenous streptokinase in acute myocardial infarction. Lancet 1985;11:842–47.

This was a randomized study of intravenous rt-PA or STK in 129 patients evaluated within 6 hours of the onset of pain. Patency at 90 minutes was significantly higher in patients treated with rt-PA (70% vs 55%). Average time to therapy was about 3 hours.

9 GAUS (German activator urokinase study). Neuhaus KL, Tebbe U, Gottwik M, *et al*. Intravenous recombinant tissue plasminogen activator (rt-PA) and urokinase in acute myocardial infarction: Results. J Am Coll Cardiol 1988;12:581–87.

This was a single-blind trial of 246 patients randomly treated with rt-PA or intravenous UK. Infarct artery patency 90 minutes after initiation of therapy was similar in the two groups (69% vs 66%). Repeat catheterization 24 hours after treatment showed less reocclusion with UK than with rt-PA (6.5% vs 14.8%). No data were provided about symptoms with reocclusion.

10 TAPS (rt-PA vs APSAC patency study) (Unpublished data).

This was a randomized trial of 195 patients comparing intravenous rt-PA and APSAC. Patients were treated on average <3 hours after onset of pain. Ninety minute infarct artery patency was 85% with rt-PA and 70% with APSAC. Repeat catheterization 24–48 hours after treatment showed patency rates of 85% with rt-PA and 92% with APSAC. Reocclusion occurred in 18 patients treated with rt-PA and only three treated with APSAC.

11 PAIMS (Plasminogen activator Italian multicenter study). Magnani B, for the PAIMS Investigators. Comparison of intravenous recombinant single-chain human tissue-type plasminogen activator (rt-PA) with intravenous streptokinase in acute myocardial infarction. J Am Coll Cardiol 1989;13:19–26.

This random trial of 171 patients with acute MI <3 hours old compared rt-PA and STK. Noninvasive signs of reperfusion (abrupt improvement in chest pain, reduced ST segments, and rapid initial increase in serum CK-MB) were observed in 79% of patients in each drug group. Follow-up cardiac catheterization 3–5 days later showed patent infarct arteries in 81% of patients treated with rt-PA and 74% of those treated with STK (p = NS). STK reduced serum plasma fibrinogen level to <1 g/liter in 87% of patients compared with just 7% of those treated with rt-PA.

12 TEAM-2 (Second trial of anistreplase in acute myocardial infarction). Anderson JL, Sorensen SG, Moreno FL, *et al*. Multicenter patency trial of intravenous anistreplase compared with streptokinase in acute myocardial infarction. Circulation 1991; 83:126–40.

This was a study of 370 patients with ST segment elevation MI who could be treated within 4 hours of symptoms. Patients were randomly treated with APSAC or STK. The endpoint, infarct artery patency at 1½–4 hours after onset of thrombolytic therapy, was comparable in the two drug groups (72% and 73%). The infarct arteries tended to look better (possibly less residual thrombus) with APSAC therapy. Safety of the two agents was comparable.

13 TEAM-3 trial (Third trial of anistreplase in acute myocardial infarction). Anderson JL, Sorensen SG, Karagounis L. A double-blind, randomized comparison of antistreplase and alteplase in acute myocardial infarction: Coronary patency results from the TEAM-3 Study. Am J Cardiol 1991;17:152A.

This was a randomized study of 322 patients with ST segment elevation infarct who could be treated <4 hours from onset of MI. Patients were treated with APSAC or rt-PA over 3 hours and all received aspirin. The patency rate at 24 hours after therapy was similar with the two drugs (90% and 85%).

14 Hogg KJ, Gemmill JD, Burns JM, *et al*. Angiographic patency study of anistreplase versus streptokinase in acute myocardial infarction. Lancet 1990;335:254–58.

This was a double-blind randomized trial of 128 patients comparing APSAC and STK. Angiographic infarct artery patency at 90 minutes was 55% and 53% with the two drugs, respectively. At 24 hours, patency of the infarct artery was 81% and 88%. There was just one early reocclusion (within 24 hours) in each treatment group.

15 Anderson JL, Rothbard RL, Hackworthy RA, *et al*. Multicenter reperfusion trial of intravenous anisoylated plasminogen streptokinase activator complex (APSAC) in acute myocardial infarction: Controlled comparison with intracoronary streptokinase. J Am Coll Cardiol 1988;11:1153–63.

This was a randomized study of 240 patients treated <6 hours from onset of MI and comparing intravenous APSAC and intra-coronary STK. All patients received heparin. A patent infarct artery at 90 minutes was found in 51% of APSAC and 60% of intracoronary STK patients (who had angiography earlier, at 60 minutes). The two regimens were considered equally safe and effective.

16 Dutch Invasive Reperfusion Study Group. Bonnier HJ, Visser RF, Klomps HC, *et al.* Comparison of intravenous anisoylated plasminogen streptokinase activator complex and intracoronary streptokinase in acute myocardial infarction. Am J Cardiol 1988; 62:25–30.

A randomized trial of 85 patients comparing intravenous APSAC and intracoronary STK. Reperfusion was achieved in 64% of APSAC and 67% of intracoronary STK treated patients. Mean time to reperfusion was 45 minutes for each drug. Slightly more reocclusion over 24 hours was noted in intracoronary STK patients.

17 KAMIT (Kentucky acute myocardial infarction trial group). Grines CL, Nissen SE, Booth DC, *et al.* A prospective, ran-domized trial comparing combination half-dose tissue-type plas-minogen activator and streptokinase with full-dose tissue-type plasminogen activator. Circulation 1991;84:540–49.

This was a randomized study of 216 patients within 6 hours of MI that compared half-dose rt-PA (50 mg) plus STK (1.5 ml units) to the conventional dose of rt-PA (100 mg). The endpoint was infarct artery patency at 90 minutes. Patients were on heparin and aspirin until follow-up catheterization at day 7. Combination therapy resulted in higher earlier patency (79%) than with rt-PA alone (64%, p <0.05). Both groups had emergency ("rescue") angioplasty for failed patency, and this brought the acute patency rate to 96% for both groups. Reocclusion, reinfarction, and the need for emergency surgery was less with the combination therapy group.

Combination therapy was more effective, and it was consider-ably less expensive.

Adjunctive therapy

Anticoagulation strategies

1 ISIS-2 Collaborative Group. (Tables 1.1, 1.2) Randomised trial of intravenous streptokinase, oral aspirin, both, or neither among 17 187 cases of suspected acute myocardial infarction: ISIS-2. Lancet 1988;2:349–60. Previously referenced under Trials Comparing Thrombolytic Therapy with Placebo.

This study establishes the importance of early aspirin as an agent which increases the rate of thrombolysis. Figure 8.4 (from the ISIS study) is among the most commonly reproduced in the thrombolytic therapy literature.

2 HART (Heparin–aspirin reperfusion trial). Hsia J, Hamilton WP, Kleiman N, *et al*. A comparison between heparin and low-dose aspirin as adjunctive therapy with tissue plasminogen activator for acute myocardial infarction. N Engl J Med 1990;323: 1433–37.

The 205 patients in this study were treated with rt-PA and randomly assigned to immediate and continuous intravenous heparin or immediate, then daily aspirin therapy. Coronary angiography was performed 7–24 hours after beginning rt-PA therapy. Infarct artery patency was found in 82% of patients in the heparin group, compared with just 52% in the aspirin group ($p <0.0001$). Repeat angiography was performed on day 7 and roughly 90% of patients in both groups had a patent infarct artery.

3 Bleich SD, Nichols T, Schumacher R, *et al*. The role of heparin following coronary thrombolysis with tissue plasminogen activator (t-PA). Circulation 1989;80(Suppl II):II–113.

This randomized trial treated 83 patients with rt-PA <6 hours from onset of MI (mean 2.7 hours). They were randomized to receive intravenous heparin or no anticoagulation. Recurrent ischemia/infarction during 7 days was identical in the two groups. However, catheterization 2–3 days after MI showed infarct artery patency 71% in patients receiving rt-PA plus heparin, and 44% in those treated with rt-PA alone ($p = 0.04$). The authors stated that heparin may thus decrease the incidence of "clinically silent coronary-reocclusion" (Chapter 7).

4 SCATI (Studio Sulla Calciparina Nell'Angina E Nella Trombosi Ventricolare Nell'Infarto Group). Randomised controlled trial of subcutaneous calcium–heparin in acute myocardial infarction. Lancet 1989;2:182–86.

Seven hundred and eleven patients with clinical and electro-cardiographic suspicion of acute MI were randomly assigned to treatment with *subcutaneous heparin* or to no adjunctive therapy; 433 patients presenting within 6 hours of chest pain also received intravenous STK. Mortality was improved by subcutaneous heparin. Patients with anterior infarction had significantly less LV mural thrombus.

5 TAMI-3 (The third trial of thrombolysis and angioplasty in myocardial infarction). Topol EJ, George BS, Kereiakes DJ, *et al*. A randomized controlled trial of intravenous tissue plasminogen activator and early intravenous heparin in acute myocardial infarction. Circulation 1989;79:281–86.

This particular TAMI trial randomly treated 134 patients with either rt-PA alone or rt-PA plus *intravenous heparin*. Infarct artery patency at 90 minutes was 79% for both groups. The implication is that intravenous heparin may not improve initial patency, which is dependent on the effectiveness of the thrombolytic agent. They imply from other studies, that the value of heparin lies with prevention of reocclusion.

Revascularization trials

6 TIMI-2 (Second study of thrombolysis in myocardial infarction). The TIMI Research Group. Immediate vs delayed catheterization and angioplasty following thrombolytic therapy for acute myocardial infarction. TIMI II A Results. JAMA 1988;260:2849–58.

Rogers WJ, Bourge RC, Papapietro SE, *et al*. Variables predictive of good functional outcome following thrombolytic therapy in the Phase II Pilot Study. Am J Cardiol 1989;63:503–12.

The TIMI Study Group. Comparison of invasive and conservative strategies after treatment with intravenous tissue plasminogen activator in acute myocardial infarction. N Engl J Med 1989;320:618–27.

Rogers WJ, Baim DS, Gore JM, *et al*. Comparison of immediate invasive, delayed invasive, and conservative strategies after tissue-type plasminogen activator. Results of the Phase II-A Trial. Circulation 1990;81:1457–76.

Roberts R, Rogers WJ, Mueller HS, *et al*. Immediate versus deferred beta-blockade following thrombolytic therapy in patients with acute myocardial infarction. Results of the Phase II-B Study. Circulation 1991;83:422–37.

This study of 3262 patients with intravenous rt-PA has been discussed at length in Chapter 7. One-half of the patients were assigned to an invasive treatment strategy consisting of coronary angiography 18–48 hours after thrombolytic therapy and prophylactic PTCA at that time. The others were treated "conservatively" and had angiography performed only if they had spontaneous or exercise-induced ischemia. Patients in the conservative wing had a predischarge exercise study that included a radionuclide angiogram. Reinfarction and death within 42 days were the primary endpoints and were similar in the two treatment groups. Predischarge ejection fraction was similar at the time of discharge and 6 weeks later. Patients in the TIMI-2A substudy had 1-year follow-up, and ejection fraction at that time was no different in conservative and invasive treatment groups.

Another subgroup was randomly treated with intravenous metoprolol given immediately and followed by oral metoprolol, or oral metoprolol begun on day 6 (TIMI-2B). Predischarge ejection fraction and mortality were similar in these two groups. However, the group receiving intravenous metoprolol had less nonfatal reinfarction and ischemia during the first 6 days.

The TIMI-2 study is widely interpreted to indicate that early angiography and revascularization are of no benefit. We take issue with this simplistic interpretation of the result for a number of reasons (Chapter 7).

7 ECSG (European Cooperative Study Group). Simoons ML, Betriu A, Col J, *et al*. Thrombolysis with tissue plasminogen activator in acute myocardial infarction: No additional benefit from immediate percutaneous coronary angioplasty. Lancet 1988; 1:197.

deBono DP. The European Cooperative Study Group Trial of intravenous recombinant tissue-type plasminogen activator (rt-PA) and conservative therapy versus rt-PA and immediate coronary angioplasty. JACC 1988;12:20–23A.

This randomized trial of 367 patients treated with rt-PA randomly assigned one-half of the patients to immediate angiography and angioplasty when feasible. Patients in this invasive wing of the study had good initial results with angioplasty, but there was a high rate of reocclusion and recurrent ischemia during the first 24 hours. Our experience agrees with these findings. We have observed that patients who have angioplasty within 24 hours of thrombolytic therapy have a higher incidence of abrupt occlusion of the artery following PTCA. It is for this reason that we delay angioplasty until 36–48 hours after thrombolytic therapy. In this study one-third of the angioplasty procedures was initiated in vessels that remained closed after treatment with rt-PA.

TAMI (thrombolysis and angioplasty in myocardial infarction) trials

This series of studies has focused upon combinations of therapies that might prove more effective than intravenous thrombolytic therapy alone. The following papers review results of each of these studies.

8 Topol EJ, Califf RM, George BS, *et al.* Insights derived from the TAMI trials. J Am Coll Cardiol 1988;12:24–31A.

This is an excellent overview of TAMI trials 1, 2, and 3, discussing the predictors of inhospital mortality, improvement of LV function, and recurrent ischemia.

9 TAMI-1 (First trial of thrombolysis and angioplasty in myocardial infarction). Topol EJ, Califf RM, George BS, *et al.* A randomized trial of immediate versus delayed elective angioplasty after intravenous tissue plasminogen activator in acute myocardial infarction. N Engl J Med 1987;317:581–88.

This study has been discussed in Chapter 7 (Fig. 7.6). It tested whether *immediate angioplasty* after intravenous thrombolytic therapy would improve patency rates. Because of the high rate of reocclusion after early angioplasty, this treatment approach was no better than one which deferred angioplasty for 5–7 days after thrombolytic therapy.

10 TAMI-2 (Second trial of thrombolysis and angioplasty in myocardial infarction). Topol EJ, Califf RM, George BS, *et al.* Coronary arterial thrombolysis with combined infusion of recombinant tissue-type plasminogen activator and urokinase in patients with acute myocardial infarction. Circulation 1988;77:1100–07.

This was a study of *combination* thrombolytic therapy using rt-PA and UK. Infarct artery patency was no higher with combination therapy. One advantage of combination therapy appeared to be a lower rate of reocclusion for patients who had "rescue angioplasty." This pilot experience led to the TAMI-5 study.

11 TAMI-3 (Third trial of thrombolysis and angioplasty in myocardial infarction). Topol EJ, George BS, Kereiakes DJ, *et al.* A randomized controlled trial of intravenous tissue plasminogen activator and early intravenous heparin in acute myocardial infarction. Circulation 1989;79:281–86.

Described above and indicating that early *heparin* therapy did not improve the rate of thrombolysis. On this basis the TAMI investigators recommended starting heparin 60–90 minutes after starting the rt-PA infusion. This approach may reduce the bleeding risk.

12 TAMI-4 (Fourth trial of thrombolysis and angioplasty in myocardial infarction). Topol EJ, Ellis SG, Califf RM, *et al.* Combined tissue-type plasminogen activator and prostacyclin therapy for acute myocardial infarction. J Am Coll Cardiol 1989;14: 877–84.

This nonrandomized trial evaluated rt-PA plus PGI_2 with rt-PA alone (25 patients in each group). Prostacyclin did not improve infarct artery patency or LV function.

13 TAMI-5 (Fifth trial of thrombolysis and angioplasty in myocardial infarction). Califf RM, Topol EJ, Stack RS, *et al.* Evaluation of combination thrombolytic therapy and timing of cardiac catheterization in acute myocardial infarction. Results of thrombolysis and angioplasty in myocardial infarction — Phase 5 randomized trial. Circulation 1991;83:1543–56.

The study compared rt-PA, rt-PA plus UK, and UK. Combination therapy was better. There was greater freedom from "any adverse event" with combination therapy (e.g., death, stroke, reinfarction, reocclusion, heart failure, or recurrent ischemia). Combination therapy caused no increase in bleeding complications. This trial also randomized patients to aggressive or conservative revascularization strategies. Aggressively treated patients had immediate angiography and PTCA if the infarct artery was occluded (rescue angioplasty). Conservatively treated patients had predischarge catheterization. Patients in the aggressive wing had fewer adverse outcomes.

14 TAMI-6 (Sixth trial of thrombolysis and angioplasty in myocardial infarction). Late therapy (Unpublished data).

This is a study of 200 patients treated with rt-PA or placebo 6–24 hours after onset of MI. Cardiac catheterization was performed within 24 hours of thrombolytic therapy. Those with occluded infarct arteries were randomly treated with rescue angioplasty. Results are not available.

15 TAMI-7 (Seventh trial of thrombolysis and angioplasty in myocardial infarction) (Unpublished data).

This is a trial of different dosing regimens for rt-PA examining front-loaded dosing and duration of drug infusion.

16 TAMI-8 (Eigth trial of thrombolysis and angioplasty in myocardial infarction). An ongoing trial of adjunctive therapy using a monoclonal antibody which inhibits platelet aggregation (Unpublished data).

17 TAMI-9 (Ninth trial of thrombolysis and angioplasty in myocardial infarction). An ongoing trial of systemic Fluisol, an oxygen-carrying compound (Unpublished data).

The central Illinois experience

1 Taylor GJ, Moses HW, Schneider JA, *et al*. Treatment of acute myocardial infarction with intracoronary infusion of streptokinase. IL Med J 1982;162:27–31.

2 Moses HW, Taylor GJ, Asali ZA, *et al.* Coronary artery spasm causing myocardial infarction. IL Med J 1983;163:265–68.

3 Taylor GJ, Mikell FL, Moses HW, *et al.* Intravenous versus intracoronary streptokinase therapy for acute myocardial infarction in community hospitals. Am J Cardiol 1984;54:256–60.

4 Taylor GJ, Mikell FL, Moses HW, *et al.* Early angiography after intravenous streptokinase demonstrates clinical efficacy. Circulation 1984;70(Suppl II):II–154.

5 Wellons HA, Schneider JA, Mikell FL, *et al.* Early operative intervention after thrombolytic therapy for acute myocardial infarction. J Vasc Surg 1985;2:186–91.

6 Mikell FL, Petrovich J, Snyder MC, *et al.* Reliability of Q-wave formation and QRS score in predicting regional and global left ventricular performance in acute myocardial infarction with successful reperfusion. Am J Cardiol 1986;57:923–26.

7 Sutton JM, Taylor GJ, Mikell FL, *et al.* Thrombolytic therapy followed by early revascularization for acute myocardial infarction. Am J Cardiol 1986;57:1227–31.

8 Petrovich JA, Schneider JA, Taylor GJ, *et al.* Early and late results of operation after thrombolytic therapy for acute myocardial infarction. J Thorac Cardiovasc Surg 1986;92:853–58.

9 Korsmeyer C, Midden AL, Taylor GJ. The nurse's role in thrombolytic therapy for acute MI. Critical Care Nurse 1987;7:22–30.

10 Epplin JJ, Wujek RA, Laughlin LD. The use of intravenous streptokinase in a rural community hospital. J Am Board Fam Pract 1988;1:87–90.

11 Petrovich JA, Wellons HA, Schneider JA, *et al.* Revascularization after thrombolytic therapy for acute myocardial infarction: An analysis of 573 patients. Ann Thorac Surg 1988;46:163–66.

12 Taylor GJ, Bourland M, Mikell FL, *et al.* Dubious reliability of Q-wave formation in predicting new regional left ventricular akinesis after coronary artery bypass grafting. Am J Cardiol 1988;62:1299–301.

13 Taylor GJ, Song A, Korsmeyer C, *et al.* Six year survival after thrombolytic for acute myocardial infarction. Circulation 1989; 80(Suppl II):520.

14 Taylor GJ, Song A, Moses HW, *et al.* The primary care physician and thrombolytic therapy for acute myocardial infarction; Comparison of intravenous streptokinase in community hospitals and tertiary referral centers. J Am Board Fam Pract 1990;3:1–6.

15 Taylor GJ, Mikell FL, Katholi RE, *et al.* Left ventricular function after transmural myocardial infarction: A blinded, randomized study comparing streptokinase and rt-PA. JACC 1991; 17:187A.

16 Taylor GJ, Mikell FL, Koester DL, *et al.* Infarct artery and lesion morphology in patients with minimal stenosis after thrombolytic therapy for acute MI. JACC 1991;17:246A.

17 Moses HW, Engelking N, Taylor GJ, *et al.* Effect of a two-year public education campaign on reducing response time of patients with symptoms of acute myocardial infarction. Am J Cardiol 1991;68:249–51.

18 Moses HW, Bartolozzi JJ, Koester DL, *et al.* Reducing delay in the emergency room in administration of thrombolytic therapy for myocardial infarction associated with ST elevation. Am J Cardiol 1991;68:251–53.

Appendix 2

Practice ECGs

These practice ECGs are from patients in the emergency department who had cardiac complaints, usually chest pain. Read the ECGs before the interpretation.

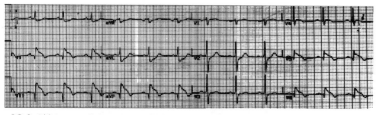

A2.1 1½ hours of chest pain, diaphoresis, and nausea. There is marked ST segment elevation in II, III, aVF, and V5-V6. There is also reciprocal ST segment depression in I and aVL. Diagnosis: inferolateral MI. This is a large MI as there is ST segment elevation in 5 leads (the size of infarction is roughly proportional to the number of leads with ST segment elevation, Chapter 2).

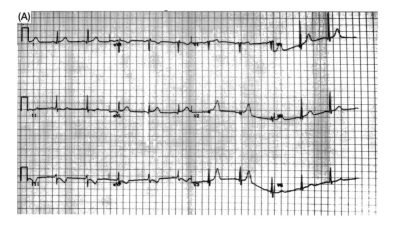

A2.2 (A) A 52-year-old man with 2 hours of chest pain. There is ST segment elevation in I and aVL. The ECG also shows ST segment depression and T wave inversion in inferior leads. Borderline ST segment elevation is noted in V2. He was treated with thrombolytic therapy for acute lateral infarction.

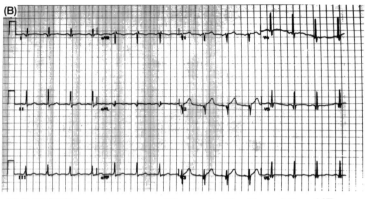

A2.2 (B) ECG the next day showed Q waves in aVL with resolution of ST segment changes.

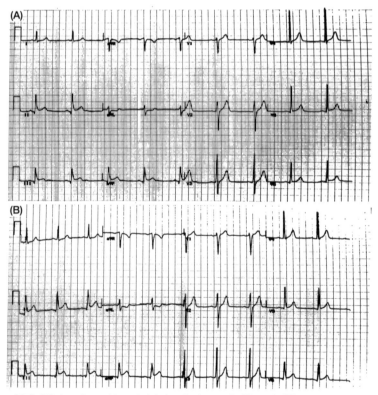

A2.3 (A) A patient with typical, ischemic chest pain. There is ST segment elevation in inferior leads with ST flattening in aVL, but the changes are not impressive. (B) The chest pain worsened. Repeat ECG 30 minutes after the first tracing shows more ST segment elevation in inferior leads and definite ST segment depression in aVL.

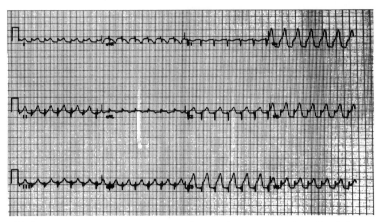

A2.4 A patient with a history of prior inferior infarction presenting with obvious acute MI. The ECG shows Q waves in inferior leads. There is ST segment elevation in anterior and lateral leads as well as sinus tachycardia (Table 6.2). This looks like a high-risk infarction. Treat with thrombolytic therapy.

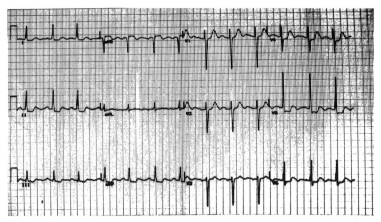

A2.5 A 70 year-old with vague chest discomfort and history of hypertension on diuretic therapy. The ECG shows ST segment depression in anterior lateral leads and prolongation of the QT interval. A review of old ECGs showed no change. Serum magnesium was 1.6 mg/dl. The ST–T changes may reflect LV hypertrophy or the electrolyte abnormality (and are thus "nonspecific").

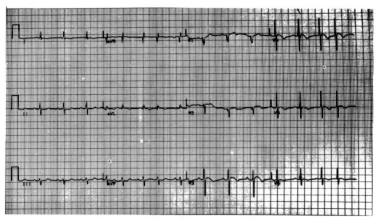

A2.6 A 77-year-old man with obstructive lung disease and chronic, atypical chest discomfort. There is minimal ST segment elevation and T wave inversion in anterior leads. The history was atypical for MI. In this case neither history nor ECG compelled us to use thrombolytic therapy. He had no CK elevation or further change in the ECG.

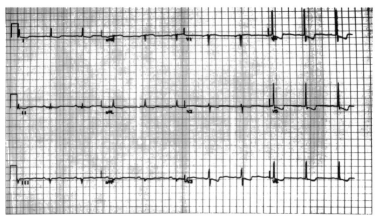

A2.7 A patient with diabetic ketoacidosis and coma. The ECG shows inferior Q waves. There are diffuse ST–T changes with a number of possible etiologies. For this reason they are considered "nonspecific." This pattern is not diagnostic for acute infarction or even ischemia. Check cardiac enzymes, but do not use thrombolytic therapy (especially with neurologic changes).

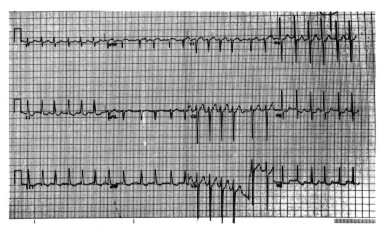

A2.8 An 80-year-old lady with dizziness. The ECG shows atrial fibrillation with a rapid ventricular rate. There is ST segment depression diffusely. These are nonspecific changes and may be related to digoxin therapy.

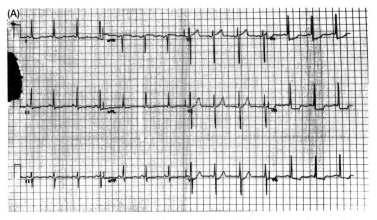

A2.9 (A) A 41-year-old man with hypertension and history suggesting unstable angina. The ECG shows ST segment depression and lateral T wave changes which could be from ischemia or LV hypertrophy. His angina was easily controlled with intravenous heparin, nitroglycerin, and beta blockers.

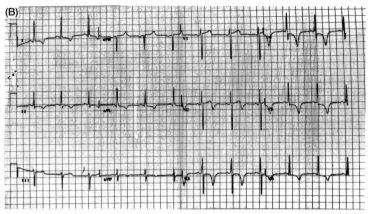

A2.9 (B) The next day the ECG shows deep and symmetrical T wave inversion in anterior and lateral leads. CK had risen to 300 iu and he was pain-free. These are the typical ECG changes of non-Q wave MI.

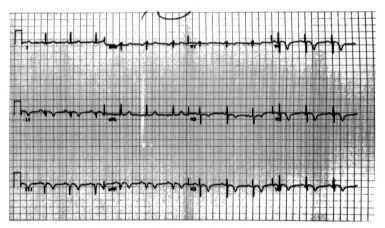

A2.10 A 66-year-old woman with history of prior MI and I hour of chest pain. The ECG shows inferior Q waves (probable prior MI), and symmetrical T wave inversion in anterior and lateral leads. The anterior T wave changes are typical for non-Q wave infarction. Her chest pain responded to sublingual nitrates and she was stable on heparin, diltiazem, and intravenous nitroglycerin. The non-Q wave MI pattern is an indication for early angiography.

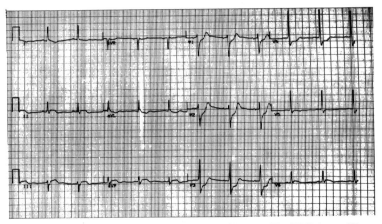

A2.11 An 82-year-old man with chest pain for 1½ hours. The ECG shows ST segment elevation in inferior leads, but it is not that dramatic. On the other hand, there was also mild ST segment elevation in V6 and he had marked, reciprocal ST segment depression in anterior leads suggesting that the inferolateral infarction was a large one. In the absence of contraindications, thrombolytic therapy was recommended.

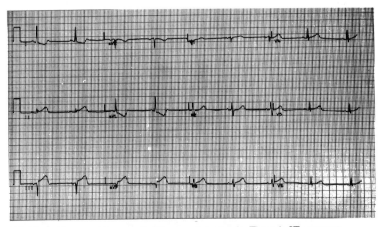

A2.12 A 68-year-old man with 3 hours of chest pain. There is ST segment elevation in inferior leads with reciprocal ST segment depression in I and aVL, indicating acute inferior MI. There are already Q waves in leads III and aVF. Is it too late to treat with thrombolytic therapy? Early appearance of Q waves does not contraindicate thrombolytic therapy particularly in a case like this where there is ongoing pain and duration of symptoms is just 3 hours.

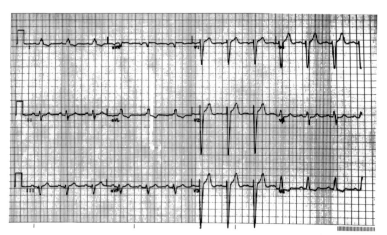

A2.13 A 63-year-old woman with atypical chest discomfort, a long history of hiatal hernia, and heartburn. The ECG shows left BBB (long QRS duration, terminal QRS forces oriented towards the left side). There is ST segment elevation in anterior leads. But with left BBB the diagnosis of acute MI cannot be made using the ECG. Based upon symptoms she was treated with antacids and had no subsequent evidence for MI.

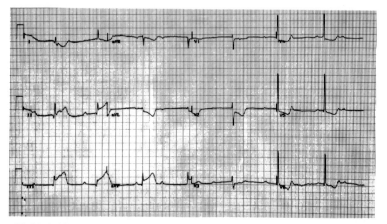

A2.14 A 60-year-old patient with chest pain and dizziness. There is ST segment elevation in inferior leads with reciprocal ST segment depression. There is also complete heart block with a junctional escape rhythm. Two hours after receiving thrombolytic therapy she had resolution of ST segment changes and heart block.

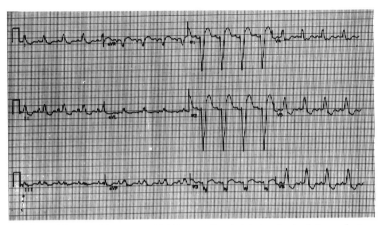

A2.15 A 72-year-old woman with 7 hours of typical, ischemic chest discomfort, nausea, diaphoresis, and hypotension. The ECG shows left BBB. Based upon symptoms, thrombolytic therapy was given for acute MI. Cardiac enzyme elevation subsequently confirmed infarction. She developed pulmonary edema, cardiogenic shock, and died the next day. A review of old ECGs showed that the left BBB was new.

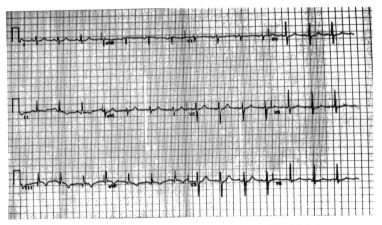

A2.16 A 49-year-old man with history of unstable angina. The ECG shows symmetrical T wave inversion in inferior leads. The changes are nonspecific, but at least they are "regional" involving just the inferior wall. They may reflect ischemia. This pattern does not indicate a need for thrombolytic therapy, and he responded to antianginal therapy.

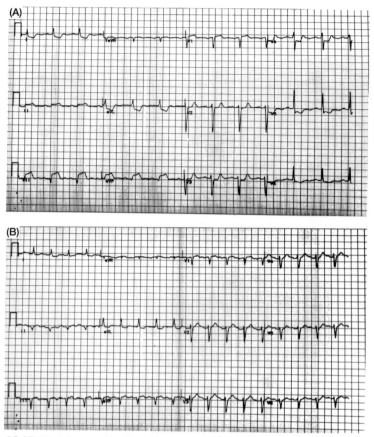

A2.17 (A) A 70-year-old man with acute inferior infarction. The ECG shows there is typical ST segment elevation in inferior leads with reciprocal lateral ST segment depression. He was treated with thrombolytic therapy 3½ hours after onset of MI. Chest pain resolved over the next 2 hours. (B) The next day he had Q waves in inferior leads with left axis deviation and poor R wave progression in anterior leads. A predischarge radionuclide angiogram showed LVEF 54% with only mild inferior hypokinesis.

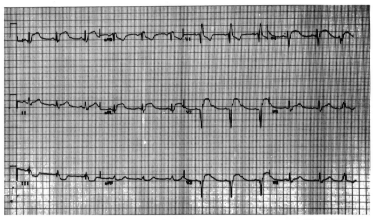

A2.18 A 71-year-old man with onset of chest pain 2 hours earlier. The ECG shows right BBB (wide QRS and rSR pattern in V1). There is ST segment elevation in anterior and lateral leads consistent with acute anterior MI. Patterns of acute infarction are not altered by right BBB.

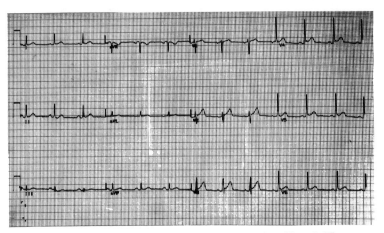

A2.19 A 26-year-old prisoner with atypical chest discomfort. There is ST segment elevation in anterior and lateral leads with minimal ST segment elevation in leads II and aVF. The changes are consistent with early repolarization.

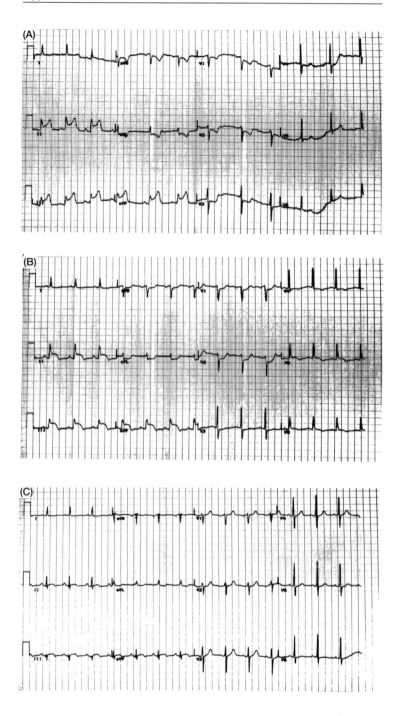

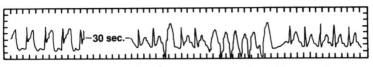

A2.21 A rhythm strip from a patient who received rt-PA 1¼ hours earlier. Over a period of 30 seconds ST segment elevation resolved, the patient had a brief run of VT and ST segments were isoelectric at the end of the arrhythmia.

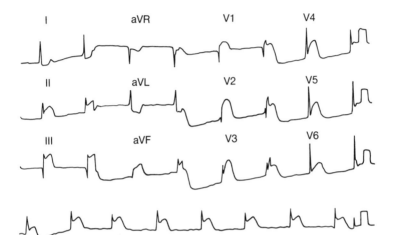

A2.22 A 69-year-old man with chest pain for 2½ hours. This ECG has dramatic ST segment elevation involving inferior and anterior leads. The global nature of ST segment elevation raises the possibility of a non-ischemic etiology (possibly pericarditis). On the other hand, there is reciprocal ST segment depression in leads I and aVL; such reciprocal changes usually are not seen with pericarditis. This patient had a clinical history consistent with acute MI and was properly treated with thrombolytic therapy. He subsequently had elevation of CK and was found to have a tight stenosis in an unusually large right coronary artery. This right coronary artery wrapped around the apex supplying a part of the anterior wall, and this may explain anterior ST-T changes. In addition, he had tight stenosis of the small anterior descending artery. Recall that the number of ECG leads with ST segment elevation is proportional to the size of the infarction. This is one of the largest acute MIs we have seen in recent years.

A2.20 (*Opposite*) Evolution of acute inferior infarction in a 66-year-old man treated with thrombolytic therapy 1 hour after onset of pain. (A) ST segment elevation in inferior leads with ST segment depression in anterolateral leads. (B) Persistent ST segment elevation but with biphasic T waves in inferior leads; this ECG was taken 30 minutes after the first. (C) Three hours later, after resolution of chest discomfort. ST segment elevation has almost resolved. There are small Q waves in inferior leads.

(A)

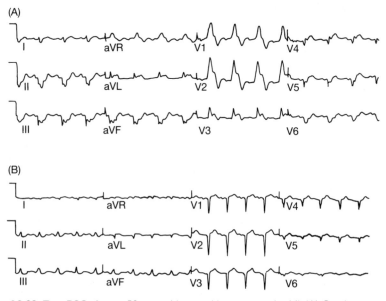

(B)

A2.23 Two ECGs from a 58-year-old man with acute anterior MI. (A) One hour after onset of pain: there is right BBB and left axis deviation ("bifascicular block") with ST segment elevation V1–4. (B) Three hours later after resolution of chest pain. The conduction abnormality has resolved as has ST segment elevation. There are Q waves V1–5. We commonly see resolution of ischemia induced conduction disturbances (AV nodal and intraventricular) with reperfusion.

Index

Page numbers in *italics* indicate an illustration separated from its text. For abbreviations see p. xi.